Stahl's Self-Assessment Examination in Psychiatry
Multiple Choice Questions for Clinicians

Third Edition

Stephen M. Stahl

*Adjunct Professor of Psychiatry
at the University of California at San Diego,
San Diego, California, USA and
Honorary Visiting Senior Fellow in Psychiatry
at the University of Cambridge, Cambridge, UK*

Editorial Assistant
Meghan M. Grady

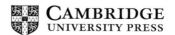
CAMBRIDGE
UNIVERSITY PRESS

CAMBRIDGE
UNIVERSITY PRESS

University Printing House, Cambridge CB2 8BS, United Kingdom

One Liberty Plaza, 20th Floor, New York, NY 10006, USA

477 Williamstown Road, Port Melbourne, VIC 3207, Australia

314–321, 3rd Floor, Plot 3, Splendor Forum, Jasola District Centre, New Delhi – 110025, India

79 Anson Road, #06–04/06, Singapore 079906

Cambridge University Press is part of the University of Cambridge.

It furthers the University's mission by disseminating knowledge in the pursuit of education, learning, and research at the highest international levels of excellence.

www.cambridge.org
Information on this title: www.cambridge.org/9781108710022
DOI: 10.1017/9781108590570

© Neuroscience Education Institute 2019

First published 2012
Second edition 2016
Third edition 2019

Printed in the United Kingdom by TJ International Ltd. Padstow Cornwall

A catalogue record for this publication is available from the British Library.

Library of Congress Cataloging-in-Publication Data
Names: Stahl, Stephen M., 1951– author.
Title: Stahl's self-assessment examination in psychiatry : multiple choice
  questions for clinicians / Stephen M. Stahl ; editorial assistant, Meghan M. Grady.
Other titles: Self-assessment examination in psychiatry
Description: Third edition. | Cambridge, United Kingdom ; New York, NY :
  Cambridge University Press, 2019. | Includes index.
Identifiers: LCCN 2018042772 | ISBN 9781108710022 (paperback)
Subjects: | MESH: Mental Disorders | Nervous System Physiological Phenomena |
  Psychiatry – methods | Examination Questions
Classification: LCC RC457 | NLM WM 18.2 | DDC 616.890076–dc23
LC record available at https://lccn.loc.gov/2018042772

ISBN 978-1-108-71002-2 Paperback

CONTENTS

INTRODUCTION/PREFACE

As many readers know, *Essential Psychopharmacology* started in 1996 as a textbook (currently in its fourth edition) on **how psychotropic drugs work** and then expanded to a companion *Prescriber's Guide* in 2005 (currently in its sixth edition) on **how to prescribe psychotropic drugs**. In 2008, a website was added (*stahlonline.org*) with both of these books available online in combination with several more, including an *Illustrated* series of several books covering specialty topics in psychopharmacology. In 2011 a case book was added, called *Case Studies: Stahl's Essential Psychopharmacology* that shows **how to apply the concepts** presented in these previous books **to real patients in a clinical practice setting**. Now comes a comprehensive set of questions and answers that we call *Stahl's Self-Assessment Examination in Psychiatry: Multiple Choice Questions for Clinicians*, designed to be integrated into the suite of our mental health/psychopharmacology books and products in the manner that I will explain here.

Why a question book?

Classically, test questions are used to measure learning, and the questions in this new book can certainly be used in this traditional manner, both by teachers and by students, and especially in combination with the companion textbook in this suite of educational products, *Stahl's Essential Psychopharmacology*. That is, teachers may wish to test student learning following their lectures on these topics by utilizing these questions and answers as part of a final examination. Also, readers not taking a formal course may wish to quiz themselves after studying specific topics in the specific chapters of the textbook. The reader will also note that documentation of the answers to each question in this book refers the reader back to the specific section of the textbook where that answer can be found and explained in great detail; outside references for the answers to the questions in the book are also provided.

Do questions just document learning?

For the modern self-directed learner, questions do much more than just document learning; they can also provide beacons for what needs to be studied and the motivation for doing that even before you read a textbook. Thus, questions are also tools for pre-study self-assessment. If you want to know whether you have already mastered a certain area of psychopharmacology, you can ask yourself these self-assessment questions BEFORE you review any specific area in the field. Many reading a textbook of psychopharmacology are not novices, but lifelong learners, and are likely to have areas of strength as well as areas of weakness. Getting correct answers will show you that a specific area is already well understood. On the other hand, getting lots of incorrect answers not only informs the self-motivated learner that a specific area needs further study, but can provide the motivation for that learner to fill in the gaps. Failure can be a powerful focuser for what to study and an energizing motivator for why to study.

"Adults don't want answers to questions they have not asked"

The truth of this old saying is that taking a test AFTER study tends to feel like being forced to answer questions that the teacher has asked. However, modern readers with the mind-set of a self-directed learner want to focus on gaps in their knowledge, so looking at these same questions PRIOR to study is a way of asking the questions of yourself and thus owning them and their answers.

What is a "knowledge sandwich?"

Ideally, self-directed learners organize their study as a "knowledge sandwich" of meaty information lying between two slices of questions. The questions in this book can be the first slice of questioning, followed by consuming the "meat" of the subject material in any textbook, including *Stahl's Essential Psychopharmacology*, or if you prefer, from a lecture, course (such as the integrated Neuroscience Education Institute's annual Psychopharmacology Congress), journal article, whatever. At the end of studying, another slice of testing shows whether learning has occurred, and whether performance has improved. You can utilize, for example, the continuing medical education (CME) tests that accompanies *Stahl's Essential Psychopharmacology* to test yourself after studying and document your learning (available at *neiglobal.com*). The rationale for this

Introduction/Preface

instructional design is also discussed in another one of our books, *Best Practices in Medical Teaching*, published in 2011. The self-assessment questions, additional "meaty" content on all the subject areas, plus posttests are also available as the "Master Psychopharmacology Program" at *neiglobal.com* for those who prefer online learning rather than a textbook.

Recertification/maintenance of certification by the American Board of Psychiatry and Neurology (ABPN)

Utilizing self-assessment questions as the first "slice" of the learning "sandwich" is not just theoretical, but is gaining prominence among expert educators these days, and indeed is now part of the requirements for maintenance of certification (MOC) in a medical specialty in the USA, including by the ABPN, which has accepted the questions in this book not only for ABPN CME requirements but also for their SA/self-assessment activity requirement, a sort of pretest.

Is your learning unforgettable?

Finally, and perhaps most importantly, tests prevent forgetting. Thus, the self-assessment questions here actually create long-term remembering, and do not just document that initial learning has occurred. It is a sorry fact that learning that occurs following one exposure/reading of material is rapidly forgotten. We have discussed this in the accompanying book in this series *Best Practices in Medical Teaching*. Perhaps 50% of what you learn after a single exposure to new, complex information is forgotten in 3–8 days, with some studies suggesting that little or nothing is remembered in 2 months! Exposing yourself to new material over time in bite-sized chunks and encountering the material again at a later time leads to more retention of information than does learning in a large bolus in a single setting, a concept sometimes called interval learning or spaced learning. Research has shown that when the re-exposure is done not as a review of the same material in the same manner, but as a test, retention is much enhanced. This results in the most efficient way of learning because the initial encoding (reading the material or hearing the lecture the first time) is consolidated for long-term retention much more effectively and completely if the re-exposure is in the form of questions. Thus, questions help you remember, and we hope that you utilize this book to maximize the efficiency of your learning to leverage the time you are able to put into your professional development.

How do you use this book?

To use this book, simply look on every right-hand page where you will see the question appear with a multiple choice format for the answer. Read the question, answer the question either in your head, on the page, or on another piece of paper. Then, turn the page and on the left hand will appear not only the correct answer, but also an explanation of why the correct answer is correct, why the incorrect answers are incorrect, and references that document the correct answers, both in the companion textbook *Stahl's Essential Psychopharmacology* and elsewhere. The reader will also see at this time what peers who have already taken this test thought was the correct answer. While taking a test, the examinee is usually curious about how (s)he is doing, how many peers get a question right, and, if the wrong answer was selected, how many peers also selected that answer wrongly. Such information can provide motivation, either as reinforcement for correct answers (yes!) or to drive the reader to understand the correct answer and never to feel the sting of missing that question again (ouch!).

So, it is with the greatest wishes for your successful journey throughout psychiatry and psychopharmacology that I present this question book to you as one of the tools for your professional development, as well as for your fascination, learning, and remembering!

Stephen M. Stahl, MD, PhD

In memory of Daniel X. Freedman, mentor, colleague, and scientific father.

CME INFORMATION

Release/expiration dates

Released: October, 2018

CME credit expires: December 31, 2020

Overview

These case-based questions, divided into 10 core areas of psychiatry, will help you identify areas in which you need further study. Each question is followed by an explanation of the answer choices and a list of suggested reference materials (recommended resources).

Learning objectives

After completing the entire book, you should be better able to:

- Diagnose patients presenting with psychiatric symptoms using evidence-based standards

- Optimize the use of available psychiatric treatments to improve patient outcomes

- Integrate recent advances in diagnostic and treatment strategies into clinical practice

Accreditation and credit designation statements

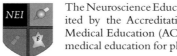

The Neuroscience Education Institute (NEI) is accredited by the Accreditation Council for Continuing Medical Education (ACCME) to provide continuing medical education for physicians.

NEI designates this enduring material for a maximum of 16.0 *AMA PRA Category 1 Credits*™. Physicians should claim only the credit commensurate with the extent of their participation in the activity. A posttest score of 70% or higher is required to receive CME credit.

The American Society for the Advancement of Pharmacotherapy (ASAP), Division 55 of the American Psychological Association, is approved by the American Psychological Association to sponsor continuing education for psychologists. ASAP maintains responsibility for this program and its content.

The American Society for the Advancement of Pharmacotherapy designates this program for 16.0 CE credits for psychologists.

Nurses and **Physician Assistants**: for all of your CE requirements for recertification, the ANCC and NCCPA will accept *AMA PRA Category 1 Credits*™ from organizations accredited by the ACCME. The content of this activity pertains to pharmacology and is worth 16.0 continuing education hours of pharmacotherapeutics.

A certificate of participation for completing this activity is available.

The content of this print monograph also exists as an online learning activity under the title "NEI Master Psychopharmacology Program Self-Assessments, 2018–2020 Edition."

ABPN – Maintenance of Certification (MOC)

The American Board of Psychiatry and Neurology (ABPN) has reviewed *Stahl's Self-Assessment Examination in Psychiatry: Multiple Choice Questions for Clinicians, Third Edition* enduring activity and has approved this program as part of a comprehensive lifelong learning and self-assessment program, which is mandated by the American Board of Medical Specialties (ABMS) as a necessary component of maintenance of certification. This activity awards *16.0 Self-Assessment Category 1 CME credits.*

More information about ABPN's Maintenance of Certification Program for psychiatry is available at www.abpn.com/maintain-certification

Instructions

The chapters of this book can be completed in any order. You are advised to read each question carefully, formulate an answer, and then review the answer/explanation on the following page. The estimated time for completion of the entire activity (including optional posttests and CME evaluations) is 16.0 hours.

Optional posttest and CME credit instructions

The optional posttests with CME credits are available online for a fee (waived for NEI members). For participant ease, each chapter has its own posttest and certificate. *NOTE*: the book as a whole is considered a single CME activity and credits earned must be totaled and submitted as such to other organizations.

To receive a certificate of CME credit or participation:

1. **Complete a chapter posttest**: *available only online at neiglobal.com/CME (under "Book")*

2. **Print the chapter certificate:** *if a score of 70% or more is achieved*

Questions? call 888-535-5600, or email CustomerService@neiglobal.com

Peer review

The content has been peer-reviewed by an MD specializing in psychiatry (excepting "Dementia and Cognitive Function and its Treatment," peer-reviewed by a PhD specializing in dementia) to ensure the scientific accuracy and medical relevance of information presented and its independence from commercial bias. NEI takes responsibility for the content, quality, and scientific integrity of this CME activity.

Disclosures

All individuals in a position to influence or control content are required to disclose any financial relationships. Although potential conflicts of interest are identified and resolved prior to the activity being presented, it remains for the participant to determine whether outside interests reflect a possible bias in either the exposition or the conclusions presented.

Disclosed financial relationships with conflicts of interest have been reviewed by the NEI CME Advisory Board Chair and resolved.

(From original online learning activity "NEI Master Psychopharmacology Program Self-Assessments, 2018–2020 Edition")

CME Information

Authors

Meghan M. Grady, BA
Director, Content Development, Neuroscience Education Institute, Carlsbad, CA
No financial relationships to disclose.

Elizabeth S. Lukins, BS
Medical Writer Associate, Neuroscience Education Institute, Carlsbad, CA
No financial relationships to disclose.

Debbi A. Morrissette, PhD
Adjunct Professor, Biological Sciences, Palomar College, San Marcos, CA
Senior Medical Writer, Neuroscience Education Institute, Carlsbad, CA
Editor, E-Cronicon Psychology and Psychiatry
No financial relationships to disclose.

Sabrina K. Segal, PhD
Adjunct Professor, Department of Psychology, Arizona State University, Tempe, AZ
Adjunct Professor, Department of Psychology, California State University Channel Islands, Camarillo, CA
Adjunct Professor, Biological Sciences, Palomar College, San Marcos, CA
Medical Writer, Neuroscience Education Institute, Carlsbad, CA
No financial relationships to disclose.

Peer reviewer

Donna M. Wilcock, PhD
Sweeney-Nelms Professor, Alzheimer's Disease Research Center, Sanders-Brown Center on Aging, Department of Physiology, University of Kentucky College of Medicine, Lexington, KY
Research/Grant: Lilly
Speakers Bureau: AC Immune, Alector
The remaining **Peer Reviewers** have no financial relationships to disclose.

Disclosure of off-label use

This educational activity may include discussion of unlabeled and/or investigational uses of agents that are not currently labeled for such use by the FDA. Please consult the product prescribing information for full disclosure of labeled uses.

Cultural and linguistic competency

A variety of resources addressing cultural and linguistic competency can be found at this link: nei.global/cmeregs

Providers

This activity is provided by NEI.
Additionally provided by the ASAP.

Support

This activity is supported solely by NEI.

1 BASIC NEUROSCIENCE

QUESTION ONE

An excitatory signal is received at the dendrite of a pyramidal glutamate neuron. When the signal is released from the incoming presynaptic dopaminergic axon, it is received as an inhibitory signal. However, this signal is not integrated properly with other incoming signals to that neuron. Which is the most likely site at which the error of integrating this signal with other incoming signals occurred?

A. Dendritic membrane

B. Soma

C. Axonal zone

D. Presynaptic zone

Answer to Question One

The correct answer is B.

Choice	Peer answers
Dendritic membrane	23%
Soma	45%
Axonal zone	14%
Presynaptic zone	18%

A – Incorrect. Dendritic membrane is the site of signal detection; signal integration does not occur here.

B – Correct. Soma is the site that integrates chemical encoding of signal transduction from all incoming signals; improper signal integration is most likely at this site.

C – Incorrect. Axonal zone is the site of signal propagation; signal integration does not occur here.

D – Incorrect. Presynaptic zone is the site of signal output; signal integration does not occur here.

References
Stahl SM. *Stahl's essential psychopharmacology*, fourth edition. New York, NY: Cambridge University Press; 2013. (Chapter 1)

Basic Neuroscience

QUESTION TWO

A receptor synthesized with an erroneous amino acid sequence is sent via fast anterograde transport to its axonal destination. If you want to find the original site of error, which organelle would you elect to observe?

A. Free polysome

B. Golgi apparatus

C. Mitochondria

D. Rough endoplasmic reticulum

Answer to Question Two

The correct answer is D.

Choice	Peer answers
Free polysome	4%
Golgi apparatus	12%
Mitochondria	13%
Rough endoplasmic reticulum	72%

A – Incorrect. Free polysomes, or non-membrane-bound ribosomes, are the site of peripheral protein (e.g., microtubules, neurofilaments) synthesis.

B – Incorrect. Golgi apparatus is the place to which integral proteins are sent for modification after synthesis.

C – Incorrect. Mitochondria, the cell's "powerhouses," are important energy sources to fuel cellular transport but will not reveal underlying causes of errors in protein synthesis.

D – Correct. The rough endoplasmic reticulum, or membrane-bound ribosomes, is the site of integral protein (e.g., receptors, enzymes, ion channels) synthesis; such proteins are destined for membrane insertion and travel via fast transport.

References
Stahl SM. *Stahl's essential psychopharmacology*, fourth edition. New York, NY: Cambridge University Press; 2013. (Chapter 1)

QUESTION THREE

Which of the following are involved in regulating neurotransmission via excitation–secretion coupling?

A. Voltage-sensitive sodium channels

B. Voltage-sensitive calcium channels

C. Both A and B

D. Neither A nor B

Basic Neuroscience

Answer to Question Three

The correct answer is C.

Choice	Peer answers
Voltage-sensitive sodium channels	10%
Voltage-sensitive calcium channels	15%
Both A and B	74%
Neither A nor B	1%

A – Partially correct.

B – Partially correct.

C – Correct. Propagation of an action potential to the axon terminal is mediated by voltage-sensitive sodium channels. Influx of sodium through voltage-sensitive sodium channels at the axon terminal leads to opening of voltage-sensitive calcium channels, also at the axon terminal. Influx of calcium through the open voltage-sensitive calcium channels leads to docking of synaptic vesicles and secretion of neurotransmitter into the synapse.

D – Incorrect.

References
Stahl SM. *Stahl's essential psychopharmacology*, fourth edition. New York, NY: Cambridge University Press; 2013. (Chapter 3)

QUESTION FOUR

Agonists cause ligand-gated ion channels to:

A. Open wider

B. Open for longer duration of time

C. Open more frequently

D. A and B

E. A and C

Answer to Question Four

The correct answer is C.

Choice	Peer answers
Open wider	3%
Open for longer duration of time	12%
Open more frequently	39%
A and B	32%
A and C	15%

A – Incorrect. Agonists do not cause ligand-gated receptors to open wider.

B – Incorrect. Agonists do not cause ligand-gated receptors to open for longer durations of time.

C – Correct. Agonists cause ligand-gated ion channels to open more frequently.

D – Incorrect.

E – Incorrect.

References

Stahl SM. *Stahl's essential psychopharmacology*, fourth edition. New York, NY: Cambridge University Press; 2013. (Chapter 3)

QUESTION FIVE

Presynaptic reuptake transporters are a major method of inactivation for which of the following?

A. Serotonin

B. Serotonin and GABA

C. Serotonin, GABA, and histamine

D. Serotonin, GABA, histamine, and neuropeptides

Answer to Question Five

The correct answer is B.

Choice	Peer answers
Serotonin	35%
Serotonin and GABA	49%
Serotonin, GABA, and histamine	8%
Serotonin, GABA, histamine, and neuropeptides	8%

A – Partially correct.

B – Correct. Both monoamines such as serotonin and amino acid neurotransmitters such as GABA are inactivated primarily via presynaptic transporters.

C – Incorrect. Histamine does not have a known presynaptic reuptake transporter and is instead inactivated via enzymatic degradation.

D – Incorrect. Histamine and neuropeptides do not have known presynaptic reuptake transporters. Histamine is inactivated enzymatically and neuropeptides are inactivated by diffusion, sequestration, and enzymatic destruction.

References
Stahl SM. *Stahl's essential psychopharmacology*, fourth edition. New York, NY: Cambridge University Press; 2013. (Chapter 2)

QUESTION SIX

A neuron is infected with a toxin and causes a rather sudden inflammatory reaction. You detect a high concentration of cytokines in the surrounding area. Which process has taken place?

A. Necrosis

B. Synaptogenesis

C. Excitotoxicity

D. Apoptosis

E. Neurogenesis

Basic Neuroscience

Answer to Question Six

The correct answer is A.

Choice	Peer answers
Necrosis	50%
Synaptogenesis	1%
Excitotoxicity	20%
Apoptosis	27%
Neurogenesis	2%

A – Correct. Necrosis is the neural selection process in which a cell is poisoned, suffocated, or otherwise destroyed by a toxin, after which the cell explodes and causes an inflammatory reaction.

B – Incorrect. Synaptogenesis is the process of forming synapses.

C – Incorrect. Excitotoxicity is a process of synaptic damage from "over-excitation," excessive amounts of which can result in cell death.

D – Incorrect. Apoptosis is triggered by a cell's own genetic machinery, causing the cell to just "fade away." The more caustic inflammatory response from cell death is associated with the neural selection process of necrosis. Cells that commit suicide (apoptosis) die in a more benign manner than when they are the victims of homicide (necrosis).

E – Incorrect. Neurogenesis is the process of forming neurons.

References

Stahl SM. *Stahl's essential psychopharmacology*, fourth edition. New York, NY: Cambridge University Press; 2013. (Chapter 1)

QUESTION SEVEN

Communication between human central nervous system (CNS) neurons at synapses is:

A. Chemical

B. Electrical

C. Both A and B

D. Neither A nor B

Answer to Question Seven

The correct answer is A.

Choice	Peer answers
Chemical	60%
Electrical	3%
Both A and B	37%
Neither A nor B	0%

A – Correct. The communication between neurons at synapses is mediated by neurotransmitter molecules and is therefore chemical.

B – Incorrect. Although electrical communication occurs within neurons during the propagation of an action potential, communication at synapses is chemical.

C – Incorrect.

D – Incorrect.

References
Stahl SM. *Stahl's essential psychopharmacology*, fourth edition. New York, NY: Cambridge University Press; 2013. (Chapter 1)

QUESTION EIGHT

A serotonin molecule binds to a 5HT2A receptor causing electrical impulses to be sent down a GABA neuron's axon terminal, eventually releasing GABA to the GABA-A receptor of its postsynaptic neuron. Which type of neurotransmission does this describe?

A. Classic synaptic neurotransmission

B. Retrograde neurotransmission

C. Volume neurotransmission

D. Signal transduction cascade

Answer to Question Eight

The correct answer is A.

Choice	Peer answers
Classic synaptic neurotransmission	76%
Retrograde neurotransmission	5%
Volume neurotransmission	1%
Signal transduction cascade	17%

A – Correct. Classic synaptic neurotransmission is the most common and well-known process of neurotransmission. It involves the anterograde transduction of a chemical signal to electrical impulses and back to chemical signals for the next neuron.

B – Incorrect. Retrograde neurotransmission is the "reverse" neurotransmission process in which a postsynaptic neuron communicates with a presynaptic neuron.

C – Incorrect. Volume neurotransmission is the process of neurotransmission without a synapse, which is also called nonsynaptic diffusion.

D – Incorrect. Signal transduction cascade is the larger process of neurocommunication that involves long strings of chemical and ionic signals.

References

Stahl SM. *Stahl's essential psychopharmacology*, fourth edition. New York, NY: Cambridge University Press; 2013. (Chapter 1)

QUESTION NINE

A receptor with four transmembrane regions changes conformation as GABA binds. Which system is this process describing?

A. Presynaptic transporter

B. Ligand–gated ion channel

C. Voltage-sensitive ion channel

Answer to Question Nine

The correct answer is B.

Choice	Peer answers
Presynaptic transporter	7%
Ligand-gated ion channel	89%
Voltage-sensitive ion channel	5%

A – Incorrect. Presynaptic transporters are 12-transmembrane region transporters that bind to neurotransmitters to transport them across the presynaptic membrane.

B – Correct. Ligand-gated ion channels are four-transmembrane region ion channels that open and close under instruction from bound neurotransmitters.

C – Incorrect. Voltage-sensitive ion channels are six-transmembrane region ion channels that open and close under instruction from charges or voltages as determined by ion flow.

References
Stahl SM. *Stahl's essential psychopharmacology*, fourth edition. New York, NY: Cambridge University Press; 2013. (Chapters 3)

QUESTION TEN

The direct role of transcription factors is to:

A. Cause neurotransmitter release

B. Influence gene expression

C. Synthesize enzymes

D. Trigger signal transduction cascades

Answer to Question Ten

The correct answer is B.

Choice	Peer answers
Cause neurotransmitter release	1%
Influence gene expression	83%
Synthesize enzymes	11%
Trigger signal transduction cascades	5%

A – Incorrect. Transcription factors do not directly cause neurotransmitter release.

B – Correct. Transcription factors are proteins that bind to promoter sequences of DNA to turn gene expression on and off.

C – Incorrect. Transcription factors do not directly cause enzyme synthesis.

D – Incorrect. Transcription factors do not directly trigger signal transduction cascades.

References

Stahl SM. *Stahl's essential psychopharmacology*, fourth edition. New York, NY: Cambridge University Press; 2013. (Chapter 1)

Basic Neuroscience

QUESTION ELEVEN

Which of the following is the most likely impetus for upregulation of D2 receptors on a striatal dopamine neuron?

A. A bound receptor is taken out of circulation

B. A new receptor is bound and put to use

C. A D2 agonist persistently binds to the receptor

D. A D2 antagonist persistently binds to the receptor

Answer to Question Eleven

The correct answer is D.

Choice	Peer answers
A bound receptor is taken out of circulation	1%
A new receptor is bound and put to use	1%
A D2 agonist persistently binds to the receptor	22%
A D2 antagonist persistently binds to the receptor	75%

A – Incorrect. A bound receptor is usually taken out of circulation when the neuron wants to decrease, not increase, the number of receptors.

B – Incorrect. A new receptor being bound and put to use is a result, not an impetus, of upregulation.

C – Incorrect. Agonists can mimic neurotransmitter actions, potentially signaling the neuron to downregulate synthesis of that receptor type.

D – Correct. Antagonists can oppose neurotransmitter actions, potentially signaling the neuron to upregulate synthesis of that receptor type.

References

Stahl SM. *Stahl's essential psychopharmacology*, fourth edition. New York, NY: Cambridge University Press; 2013. (Chapters 3, 5)

QUESTION TWELVE

What is the correct order and direction of ion flow into and out of a neuron experiencing an action potential?

A. Na^+ in, K^+ out, Ca^{2+} in

B. Ca^{2+} in, K^+ out, Na^+ in

C. K^+ in, Na^+ in, Ca^{2+} in

D. Na^+ in, Ca^{2+} in, K^+ out

E. Ca^{2+} in, Na^+ out, K^+ out

F. K^+ in, Ca^{2+} in, Na^+ out

Answer to Question Twelve

The correct answer is D.

Choice	Peer answers
Na+ in, K+ out, Ca2+ in	39%
Ca2+ in, K+ out, Na+ in	3%
K+ in, Na+ in, Ca2+ in	1%
Na+ in, Ca2+ in, K+ out	50%
Ca2+ in, Na+ out, K+ out	4%
K+ in, Ca2+ in, Na+ out	4%

A, B, C, E, and F – Incorrect.

D – Correct. Sodium enters the cell followed by an influx of calcium; potassium exits the neuron at the end of the action potential, restoring the baseline electrical charge in the cell.

References

Stahl SM. *Stahl's essential psychopharmacology*, fourth edition. New York, NY: Cambridge University Press; 2013. (Chapter 3)

QUESTION THIRTEEN

What are the molecular mechanisms of epigenetics?

A. Molecular gates are opened by acetylation and/or demethylation of histones, allowing transcription factors access to genes, thus activating them

B. Molecular gates are opened by deacetylation and/or methylation, allowing transcription factors access to genes, thus activating them

C. Molecular gates are closed by deacetylation and/or methylation, preventing access of transcription factors to genes, thus silencing them.

D. A and C

Answer to Question Thirteen

The correct answer is D.

Choice	Peer answers
Molecular gates are opened by acetylation and/or demethylation of histones, allowing transcription factors access to genes, thus activating them	19%
Molecular gates are opened by deacetylation and/or methylation, allowing transcription factors access to genes, thus activating them	12%
Molecular gates are closed by deacetylation and/or methylation, preventing access of transcription factors to genes, thus silencing them	3%
A and C	66%

A – Partially correct. Epigenetic control over whether genes are activated (i.e., expressed) or silenced is achieved by the modification of chromatin. Acetylation and demethylation of histones decompress the chromatin, opening the molecular gates, allowing transcription factors to get to the promoter regions of genes and activate them.

B – Incorrect.

C – Partially correct. Methylation of histones can silence genes, whereas demethylation of histones can activate genes. Methylation of DNA can result in deacetylation of histones by activating enzymes called histone deacetylases (HDACs). Deacetylation of histones also has a silencing effect on gene expression. Methylation and deacetylation compress chromatin, closing the molecular gates, which prevents the transcription factors from accessing the promoter regions that activate genes, thus silencing them.

D – Correct.

References

Stahl SM. *Stahl's essential psychopharmacology*, fourth edition. New York, NY: Cambridge University Press; 2013. (Chapter 1)

QUESTION FOURTEEN

N-methyl-D-aspartate (NMDA) receptors are activated by:

A. Glutamate

B. Glycine

C. Depolarization

D. Glutamate and glycine

E. Glutamate and depolarization

F. Glycine and depolarization

G. Glutamate, glycine, and depolarization

Answer to Question Fourteen

The correct answer is G.

Choice	Peer answers
Glutamate	22%
Glycine	1%
Depolarization	1%
Glutamate and glycine	17%
Glutamate and depolarization	13%
Glycine and depolarization	1%
Glutamate, glycine, and depolarization	45%

A–F – Incorrect.

G – Correct. N-methyl-D-aspartate (NMDA) receptors are ligand-gated ion channels that regulate excitatory postsynaptic neurotransmission triggered by glutamate. In the resting state, NMDA receptors are blocked by magnesium, which plugs the calcium channel. Opening of NMDA glutamate receptors requires the presence of both glutamate and glycine, each of which bind to a different site on the receptor. When magnesium is also bound and the membrane is not depolarized, it prevents the effects of glutamate and glycine and thus does not allow the ion channel to open. In order for the channel to open and permit calcium entry, depolarization must remove magnesium while both glutamate and glycine are bound to their sites.

References

Stahl SM. *Stahl's essential psychopharmacology*, fourth edition. New York, NY: Cambridge University Press; 2013. (Chapter 4)

Basic Neuroscience

QUESTION FIFTEEN

Neurogenesis has recently been discovered to occur in adults:

A. Only in the dentate gyrus of the hippocampus

B. In the dentate gyrus of the hippocampus and in the olfactory bulb

C. In the dentate gyrus of the hippocampus, in the olfactory bulb, and in the lateral nucleus of the amygdala

D. Throughout the brain

Basic Neuroscience

Answer to Question Fifteen

The correct answer is B.

Choice	Peer answers
Only in the dentate gyrus of the hippocampus	7%
In the dentate gyrus of the hippocampus and in the olfactory bulb	39%
In the dentate gyrus of the hippocampus, in the olfactory bulb, and in the lateral nucleus of the amygdala	16%
Throughout the brain	38%

A – Incorrect. Although adult neurogenesis does occur in the dentate gyrus, this is not the only brain region where adult neurogenesis occurs.

B – Correct. Adult neurogenesis occurs in both the dentate gyrus of the hippocampus and in the olfactory bulb.

C – Incorrect. Although adult neurogenesis occurs in both the dentate gyrus and the olfactory bulb, there is no evidence that adult neurogenesis occurs in the lateral nucleus of the amygdala.

D – Incorrect. Adult neurogenesis occurs only in the dentate gyrus and in the olfactory bulb.

References

Hagg T. Molecular regulation of adult CNS neurogenesis: an integrated view. *Trends Neurosci* 2005;28(11):589–95.

Ming GL, Song H. Adult neurogenesis in the mammalian brain: significant answers and significant questions. *Neuron* 2011;70(4):687–702.

QUESTION SIXTEEN

A signal transduction cascade passes its message from an extracellular first messenger to an intracellular second messenger. In the case of the G-protein-linked systems, the second messenger is a:

A. Ion

B. Hormone

C. Chemical

D. Kinase enzyme

Answer to Question Sixteen

The correct answer is C.

Choice	Peer answers
Ion	12%
Hormone	6%
Chemical	44%
Kinase enzyme	38%

A – Incorrect. For an ion-channel-linked system, the second messenger can be an ion, such as calcium. For a G-protein-linked system, the second messenger is a chemical.

B – Incorrect. For some hormone-linked systems, a second messenger is formed when a hormone finds its receptor in the cytoplasm and binds to it to form a hormone–nuclear receptor complex. For a G-protein-linked system, the second messenger is a chemical.

C – Correct. For a G-protein-linked system, the second messenger is a chemical. The four key elements to the G-protein second-messenger system are: (1) the first messenger neurotransmitter; (2) a receptor for the neurotransmitter that belongs to the receptor superfamily in which all have the structure of seven transmembrane regions; (3) a G-protein capable of binding both to certain conformations of the neurotransmitter receptor and to the enzyme system that can synthesize the second messenger; (4) the enzyme system itself for the second messenger.

D – Incorrect. For neurotrophins, a complex set of second messengers exist, including proteins that are kinase enzymes. For a G-protein-linked system, the second messenger is a chemical.

References

Stahl SM. *Stahl's essential psychopharmacology*, fourth edition. New York, NY: Cambridge University Press; 2013. (Chapter 2)

CHAPTER PEER COMPARISON

For the Basic Neuroscience section, the correct answer was selected 60% of the time.

2 PSYCHOSIS AND SCHIZOPHRENIA AND ANTIPSYCHOTICS

QUESTION ONE

A 24-year-old male initially presents with acute auditory hallucinations and is treated with medication. Four days later he arrives at your office for evaluation. You observe that he is neatly dressed, avoids eye contact, and gives very short answers to your initial questions. Which of the following questions would be most beneficial for determining his degree of negative symptoms?

A. How often have you visited with friends in the past week?

B. Have the voices you've heard persisted or returned?

C. Have you ever thought about hurting yourself or someone else?

D. In the past week have you had difficulty concentrating?

Answer to Question One

The correct answer is A.

Choice	Peer answers
How often have you visited with friends in the past week?	83%
Have the voices you've heard persisted or returned?	4%
Have you ever thought about hurting yourself or someone else?	3%
In the past week have you had difficulty concentrating?	10%

A – Correct. How often have you visited with friends in the past week: This is a useful question when assessing for negative symptoms, as an important component of negative symptoms is reduced social drive.

B – Incorrect. Have the voices you've heard persisted or returned: Although this question is useful for determining the presence of positive symptoms, it is not applicable to assessment of negative symptoms.

C – Incorrect. Have you ever thought about hurting yourself or someone else: This question can help assess for risk of suicide as well as any possible aggression risk, but these are not part of the negative symptom domain.

D – Incorrect. In the past week have you had difficulty concentrating: This question is applicable to assessment for cognitive symptoms, but not for negative symptoms.

References

Stahl SM. *Stahl's essential psychopharmacology*, fourth edition. New York, NY: Cambridge University Press; 2013. (Chapter 4)

Stahl SM, Buckley PF. Negative symptoms of schizophrenia: a problem that will not go away. *Acta Psychiatr Scand* 2007;15:4–11.

QUESTION TWO

A 21-year-old man who has just been diagnosed with schizophrenia presents with his parents. He speaks with a reserved and simple language processing style; he is able to understand and relate to simple questions, but seems to get lost when the pace of the conversation between the clinician and parents accelerates. When reviewing the patient's history, what pattern of cognitive functioning prior to psychosis onset would you be most likely to find?

A. Normal cognitive functioning during premorbid and prodromal phases

B. Impaired cognitive functioning that is stable across premorbid and prodromal phases

C. Impaired cognitive functioning premorbidly with further decline during the prodromal phase

D. Progressive decline of cognitive functioning premorbidly, which stabilizes in the prodromal phase

Answer to Question Two

The correct answer is C.

Choice	Peer answers
Normal cognitive functioning during premorbid and prodromal phases	10%
Impaired cognitive functioning that is stable across premorbid and prodromal phases	7%
Impaired cognitive functioning premorbidly with further decline during the prodromal phase	73%
Progressive decline of cognitive functioning premorbidly, which stabilizes in the prodromal phase	11%

Individuals who ultimately develop schizophrenia typically exhibit a deficit in cognitive and social functioning that **begins in childhood**, with a **notable decline** in cognitive and social functioning that occurs during adolescence and precedes the onset of psychosis. This decline in cognitive functioning coincides with the neurodevelopmental period known as competitive elimination, during which extensive brain restructuring and synaptic pruning takes place.

A – Incorrect. Individuals with schizophrenia typically exhibit a history of cognitive impairment prior to psychosis onset.

B – Incorrect. Individuals with schizophrenia typically experience a decline in functioning during the prodromal phase.

C – Correct. Individuals with schizophrenia typically exhibit impaired cognitive functioning premorbidly with further decline during the prodromal phase.

D – Incorrect. Individuals with schizophrenia generally show stable cognitive functioning premorbidly, with decline not occurring until the prodromal phase.

References

Insel TR. Rethinking schizophrenia. *Nature* 2010;468:187–93.

McGorry PD, Yung AR, Bechdolf A, Amminger P. Back to the future: predicting and reshaping the course of psychotic disorder. *Arch Gen Psychiatry* 2008;65:25–7.

Neuroscience Education Institute. Why Don't Dopamine 2 Antagonists Improve Cognition in Schizophrenia? Part 1: NMDA Receptors and The Proposed Origins of Schizophrenia [Animation]. 2015.

QUESTION THREE

A 24-year-old woman is hospitalized after an altercation in which she screamed at and attacked her neighbor when he knocked on her door. Her mother reports that she has been increasingly erratic recently, with emotional outbursts and impulsive behavior. Which of the following brain regions is most likely associated with these symptoms?

A. Dorsolateral prefrontal cortex

B. Nucleus accumbens

C. Orbital frontal cortex

D. Substantia nigra

Answer to Question Three

The correct answer is C.

Choice	Peer answers
Dorsolateral prefrontal cortex	30%
Nucleus accumbens	7%
Orbital frontal cortex	62%
Substantia nigra	2%

A – Incorrect. Dorsolateral prefrontal cortex: This brain region is hypothetically associated with cognition and executive functioning, not with aggression.

B – Incorrect. Nucleus accumbens: This brain region is hypothetically associated with positive symptoms such as delusions and hallucinations. Although aggressive symptoms, such as those exhibited by this patient, often occur in conjunction with positive symptoms, they may not be localized to the nucleus accumbens.

C – Correct. Orbital frontal cortex: Aggressive symptoms such as those exhibited by this patient are hypothetically associated with impairment in impulse control, which is largely regulated by the orbital frontal cortex.

D – Incorrect. Substantia nigra: This region in the brainstem houses dopaminergic cell bodies that project to the striatum. The substantia nigra is not particularly linked to aggression.

References

Stahl SM. *Stahl's essential psychopharmacology*, fourth edition. New York, NY: Cambridge University Press; 2013. (Chapter 4)

Stahl SM, Mignon L. *Stahl's illustrated antipsychotics*, second edition. Carlsbad, CA: NEI Press; 2009. (Chapter 1)

QUESTION FOUR

A major current hypothesis for the cause of schizophrenia proposes that N-methyl-D-aspartate (NMDA) receptors may be:

A. Hypofunctional

B. Hyperfunctional

Answer to Question Four

The correct answer is A.

Choice	Peer answers
Hypofunctional	66%
Hyperfunctional	34%

A – Correct. A major current hypothesis for the cause of schizophrenia proposes that glutamate activity at *N*-methyl-D-aspartate (NMDA) receptors is **hypo**functional due to abnormalities in the formation of glutamatergic NMDA synapses during neurodevelopment.

Normally, when glutamate synapses are active, their NMDA receptors trigger an electrical phenomenon known as long-term potentiation, or LTP. LTP leads to structural and functional changes of the synapse that make neurotransmission more efficient, sometimes called "strengthening" of synapses. During pubescence and adolescence, a period known as competitive elimination occurs, with extensive synaptic pruning and restructuring. Frequently used synaptic connections with efficient NMDA neurotransmission survive, whereas infrequently used synaptic connections with less active NMDA receptors may be targets for elimination. This shaping of the brain's circuits normally allows the most critical synapses to survive, while inefficient and rarely utilized synapses are eliminated. Abnormalities in the NMDA receptor may jeopardize this essential process and increase risk for neurodevelopmental disorders such as schizophrenia.

B – Incorrect. NMDA receptors are not hypothesized to be hyperfunctional in schizophrenia.

References

Neuroscience Education Institute. Why Don't Dopamine 2 Antagonists Improve Cognition in Schizophrenia? Part 1: NMDA Receptors and The Proposed Origins of Schizophrenia [Animation]. 2015.

Neuroscience Education Institute. Why Don't Dopamine 2 Antagonists Improve Cognition in Schizophrenia? Part 2: The Hypothetical Roles of Glutamate and GABA [Animation]. 2015.

Stahl SM. *Stahl's essential psychopharmacology*, fourth edition. New York, NY: Cambridge University Press; 2013. (Chapter 4, pp. 107–114, 122)

QUESTION FIVE

Tim is a 17-year-old patient with first-onset schizophrenia. He is currently taking the antipsychotic fluphenazine but is not experiencing any relief from his positive symptoms. Lab testing reveals that Tim's fluphenazine plasma levels are low; thus, there may not be sufficient blockade of dopamine 2 receptors. In order for an antipsychotic to exert therapeutic effects, what is the minimum hypothetical threshold of D2 receptor occupancy?

A. >20%

B. >40%

C. >60%

D. >90%

Answer to Question Five

The correct answer is C.

Choice	Peer answers
>20%	3%
>40%	14%
>60%	80%
>90%	3%

A – Incorrect. With only 20% D2 receptor occupancy, it is unlikely that a pharmacologic agent will have any therapeutic effects.

B – Incorrect. With only 40% D2 receptor occupancy, it is unlikely that a pharmacologic agent will have any therapeutic effects.

C – Correct. Data indicate that 60% D2 receptor occupancy is the minimum threshold for antipsychotic efficacy.

D – Incorrect. D2 receptor occupancy of 90% is well above the hypothetical minimum threshold for antipsychotic effects, and is also above the hypothetical threshold for inducing extrapyramidal side effects.

References
Stahl SM. *Stahl's essential psychopharmacology*, fourth edition. New York, NY: Cambridge University Press; 2013. (Chapter 5)

Stahl SM. *Essential psychopharmacology, the prescriber's guide*, sixth edition. New York, NY: Cambridge University Press; 2017.

QUESTION SIX

Based on thorough evaluation of a patient and his history, his care provider intends to begin treatment with a conventional antipsychotic but has not selected a particular agent yet. Which of the following is most true about conventional antipsychotics?

A. They are very similar in therapeutic profile but differ in side-effect profile

B. They are very similar in both therapeutic and side-effect profile

C. They differ in therapeutic profile but are similar in side-effect profile

D. They differ in both therapeutic and side-effect profile

Answer to Question Six

The correct answer is A.

Choice	Peer answers
They are very similar in therapeutic profile but differ in side-effect profile	73%
They are very similar in both therapeutic and side-effect profile	11%
They differ in therapeutic profile but are similar in side-effect profile	7%
They differ in both therapeutic and side-effect profile	8%

A – Correct. Although individual effects may vary from patient to patient, in general conventional antipsychotics share the same primary mechanism of action and do not differ much in their therapeutic profiles. There are, however, differences in secondary properties, such as degree of muscarinic, histaminergic, and/or alpha adrenergic receptor antagonism, which can lead to different side-effect profiles.

B, C, and D – Incorrect.

References

Stahl SM. *Stahl's essential psychopharmacology*, fourth edition. New York, NY: Cambridge University Press; 2013. (Chapter 5)

Stahl SM. *Essential psychopharmacology, the prescriber's guide*, sixth edition. New York, NY: Cambridge University Press; 2017.

QUESTION SEVEN

A 34-year-old man is initiated on an atypical antipsychotic for the treatment of schizophrenia. The majority of atypical antipsychotics:

A. Have higher affinity for dopamine 2 receptors than for serotonin 2A receptors

B. Have higher affinity for serotonin 2A receptors than for dopamine 2 receptors

Answer to Question Seven

The correct answer is B.

Choice	Peer answers
Have higher affinity for dopamine 2 receptors than for serotonin 2A receptors	28%
Have higher affinity for serotonin 2A receptors than for dopamine 2 receptors	72%

A – Incorrect (have higher affinity for serotonin 2A receptors than for dopamine 2 receptors).

B – Correct. Because nearly all atypical antipsychotics have actions at serotonin 2A receptors, it may be beneficial to understand how stimulating or blocking these receptors can regulate dopamine release.

Serotonin neurons originate in the raphe nucleus of the brainstem and project throughout the brain, including to the cortex. They synapse there with glutamatergic pyramidal neurons, which project to the substantia nigra in the brainstem. The substantia nigra is the origin of dopaminergic neurons that project to the striatum. All serotonin 2A receptors are postsynaptic. When they are located on cortical pyramidal neurons, they are excitatory. Thus, when serotonin is released in the cortex and binds to serotonin 2A receptors on glutamatergic pyramidal neurons, this stimulates them to release glutamate in the brainstem, which in turn stimulates GABA release. GABA binds to dopaminergic neurons projecting from the substantia nigra to the striatum, inhibiting dopamine release and possibly leading to extrapyramidal side effects (EPS).

Nearly all atypical antipsychotics have an affinity for blocking serotonin 2A receptors that is equal to or greater than their affinity for blocking dopamine 2 receptors. The "pines" – clozapine, olanzapine, quetiapine, and asenapine – all bind much more potently to the serotonin 2A receptor than they do to the dopamine 2 receptor. The "dones" – risperidone, paliperidone, ziprasidone, iloperidone, and lurasidone – also bind more potently to the serotonin 2A receptor than to the dopamine 2 receptor, or show similar potency at both receptors. Aripiprazole and cariprazine bind more potently to the dopamine 2 receptor than to the serotonin 2A receptor; however, they are also partial agonists at dopamine 2 receptors. Brexpiprazole (also a dopamine 2 partial agonist) has comparable binding affinity to the dopamine 2 and serotonin 2A receptors.

References

Roth BL. Ki determinations, receptor binding profiles, agonist and/or antagonist functional data, HERG data, MDR1 data, etc. as appropriate was generously provided by the National Institute of Mental Health's Psychoactive Drug Screening Program, Contract # HHSN-271–2008-00025-C (NIMH PDSP). The NIMH PDSP is directed by Bryan L. Roth MD, PhD at the University of North Carolina at Chapel Hill and Project Officer Jamie Driscol at NIMH, Bethesda MD, USA. For experimental details please refer to the PDSP website http://pdsp.med.unc.edu.

Stahl SM. *Stahl's essential psychopharmacology*, fourth edition. New York, NY: Cambridge University Press; 2013.

Psychosis and Schizophrenia and Antipsychotics

QUESTION EIGHT

A 34-year old male recently began experiencing breast secretions while receiving perphenazine. After switching to quetiapine the secretions ceased. Which of the following is the most likely pharmacological explanation for the resolution of this side effect?

A. Dopamine 2 antagonism

B. Serotonin 2A antagonism

C. Serotonin 2C antagonism

D. Histamine 1 antagonism

Answer to Question Eight

The correct answer is B.

Choice	Peer answers
Dopamine 2 antagonism	33%
Serotonin 2A antagonism	49%
Serotonin 2C antagonism	11%
Histamine 1 antagonism	7%

A – Incorrect. Stimulation of D2 receptors inhibits prolactin release; thus a dopamine 2 antagonist such as perphenazine could increase prolactin release and potentially lead to breast secretions.

B – Correct. Stimulation of serotonin 2A receptors stimulates prolactin release. As they have opposing effects on prolactin, adding serotonin 2A antagonism to dopamine 2 antagonism results in a neutral effect on prolactin and may relieve breast secretions caused by dopamine 2 antagonism alone.

C and D – Incorrect. Although quetiapine is an antagonist at serotonin 2C and histamine 1 receptors, both of which are associated with some side effects, neither receptor type has an established role in prolactin elevation.

References

Stahl SM. *Stahl's essential psychopharmacology*, fourth edition. New York, NY: Cambridge University Press; 2013. (Chapter 5)

Stahl SM, Mignon L. *Stahl's illustrated antipsychotics*, second edition. Carlsbad, CA: NEI Press; 2009. (Chapter 2)

QUESTION NINE

Compared to aripiprazole, where do brexpiprazole and cariprazine fall on the dopamine agonist spectrum?

A. Brexpiprazole and cariprazine have less intrinsic activity/are more antagonistic than aripiprazole

B. Brexpiprazole and cariprazine have more intrinsic activity/are more of an agonist than aripiprazole

Answer to Question Nine

The correct answer is A.

Choice	Peer answers
Brexpiprazole and cariprazine have less intrinsic activity/are more antagonistic than aripiprazole	56%
Brexpiprazole and cariprazine have more intrinsic activity/are more of an agonist than aripiprazole	44%

A – Correct. Brexpiprazole and cariprazine, like aripiprazole, are partial agonists at the dopamine 2 receptor. Pharmacologically, brexpiprazole has less intrinsic activity (i.e., is less of a partial agonist and more of an antagonist) at dopamine 2 receptors than aripiprazole. Similarly, cariprazine also has less intrinsic activity at dopamine 2 receptors than aripiprazole; its activity is very similar to brexpiprazole. Cariprazine and brexpiprazole differ from each other in terms of their secondary pharmacological properties.

B – Incorrect.

References
Stahl SM. Mechanism of action of brexpiprazole: comparison with aripiprazole. *CNS Spectr* 2016;21:1–6.
Stahl SM. Mechanism of action of cariprazine. *CNS Spectr* 2016;21: 123–7.

QUESTION TEN

Frank is a 24-year-old patient recently diagnosed with schizophrenia. He is currently taking an antipsychotic, and his psychosis symptoms are reasonably well resolved. At a follow-up visit, you notice that Frank does not seem to be able to sit still; he is constantly pacing the examining room, and when he does sit down, he rocks back and forth, fidgets, and repetitively crosses and uncrosses his legs. Drug-induced akathisia is caused by:

A. Dopaminergic hypoactivity

B. Dopaminergic hyperactivity

C. The pathophysiology is not known

Answer to Question Ten

The correct answer is C.

Choice	Peer answers
Dopaminergic hypoactivity	38%
Dopaminergic hyperactivity	27%
The pathophysiology is not known	35%

Akathisia is a distressing side effect characterized by a subjective feeling of inner restlessness that prompts a need to move. It is often extraordinarily difficult for the patient to describe, in part because there are few subjective states to which it can be compared.

A – Incorrect. Dopaminergic hypoactivity has been proposed as an underlying cause of akathisia because most antipsychotics are potent antagonists at the dopamine 2 receptor, it occurs in Parkinson's disease, and similar disorders (restless legs syndrome and periodic limb movement disorder) are treated with dopamine agonists. However, there is no established direct link between parkinsonism and akathisia, and agents that cause the least extrapyramidal side effects (EPS) can still cause akathisia. In addition, other agents can also cause akathisia, including notably the selective serotonin reuptake inhibitors (SSRIs).

B – Incorrect. Akathisia has not been linked to dopamine hyperactivity.

C – Correct. The pathophysiology of akathisia is not known.

References
Lohr JB, Eidt CA, Abdulrazzaq Alfaraj A, Soliman MA. The clinical challenges of akathisia. *CNS Spectr* 2015;20:4–14.

Stahl SM, Loonen AJ. The mechanism of drug-induced akathisia. *CNS Spectr* 2011;16(1):7–10.

QUESTION ELEVEN

A 44-year-old woman with schizophrenia has developed tardive dyskinesia after taking haloperidol 15 mg/day for 2 years. Which of the following would be the most appropriate pharmacologic mechanism to manage her tardive dyskinesia?

A. Antagonism at serotonin 2A receptors

B. Antagonism of beta adrenergic receptors

C. Inhibition of vesicular monoamine transporter 2

D. Antagonism of muscarinic acetylcholine receptors

Answer to Question Eleven

The correct answer is C.

Choice	Peer answers
Antagonism at serotonin 2A receptors	17%
Antagonism of beta adrenergic receptors	7%
Inhibition of vesicular monoamine transporter 2	45%
Antagonism of muscarinic acetylcholine receptors	31%

Tardive dyskinesia is a neurological disorder characterized by repetitive involuntary movements usually associated with lower facial and distal extremity musculature. Common signs include tongue protrusion, writhing of tongue, lip smacking, chewing, blinking, and grimacing. Tardive dyskinesia will reverse in approximately one-third of patients over a 6-month period after the offending medication is discontinued. For patients who do not experience reversal of their tardive dyskinesia, there are augmentation options to treat it.

A – Incorrect. Although dopamine 2 antagonists with the additional property of serotonin 2A antagonism were initially thought to carry less risk of tardive dyskinesia, it is now known that tardive dyskinesia continues to be a potential side effect of these agents, and that any possibly reduced risk does not necessarily seem to correlate with the degree of serotonin 2A antagonism.

B – Incorrect. Beta blockers (e.g., propranolol) do not show evidence of efficacy in the treatment of tardive dyskinesia.

C – Correct. The best evidenced (including approved) medications to treat tardive dyskinesia are selective inhibitors of vesicular monoamine transporter 2 (VMAT2), which packages monoamines, including dopamine, into synaptic vesicles of presynaptic neurons in the central nervous system.

D – Incorrect. Central anticholinergic medication can improve drug-induced parkinsonism, but exacerbate or unmask tardive dyskinesia. This effect may be reversible if the anticholinergic medication is discontinued.

References

Fernandez HH, Factor SA, Hauser RA et al. Randomized controlled trial of deutetrabenazine for tardive dyskinesia: the ARM-TD study. *Neurology* 2017;88(21):-2003–10.

Hauser RA, Factor SA, Marder SR et al. KINECT 3: a phase 3 randomized, double-blind, placebo-controlled trial of valbenazine for tardive dyskinesia. *Am J Psychiatry* 2017;174(5):-476–84.

Waln O, Jankovic J. An update on tardive dyskinesia: from phenomenology to treatment. *Tremor Other Hyperkinetic Movements*, 2013;3. doi:10.7916/D88P5Z71.

Psychosis and Schizophrenia and Antipsychotics

QUESTION TWELVE

A patient who has been taking an atypical antipsychotic for 6 months has experienced a 22-pound weight gain since baseline. Which of the following pharmacologic properties most likely underlies this patient's metabolic changes?

A. Dopamine 2 antagonism

B. Serotonin 2A antagonism

C. Serotonin 2C antagonism

D. Alpha 1 adrenergic antagonism

Psychosis and Schizophrenia and Antipsychotics

Answer to Question Twelve

The correct answer is C.

Choice	Peer answers
Dopamine 2 antagonism	3%
Serotonin 2A antagonism	18%
Serotonin 2C antagonism	72%
Alpha 1 adrenergic antagonism	7%

A – Incorrect. Antagonism of dopamine 2 receptors is associated with both therapeutic and side effects, but is not linked to weight gain.

B – Incorrect. Similarly, antagonism of serotonin 2A receptors has not been linked to risk for weight gain.

C – Correct. Antagonism of serotonin 2C receptors is associated with increased risk for weight gain, perhaps in part due to stimulation of appetite regulated by the hypothalamus, and especially in combination with histamine 1 antagonism.

D – Incorrect. Antagonism of alpha 1 adrenergic receptors is associated with side effects, but is not linked to weight gain.

References

Stahl SM. *Stahl's essential psychopharmacology*, fourth edition. New York, NY: Cambridge University Press; 2013. (Chapter 5)

Stahl SM. *Essential psychopharmacology, the prescriber's guide*, sixth edition. New York, NY: Cambridge University Press; 2017.

Stahl SM, Mignon L. *Stahl's illustrated antipsychotics*, second edition. Carlsbad, CA: NEI Press; 2009. (Chapter 3)

QUESTION THIRTEEN

A 34-year-old woman with schizophrenia has been taking a therapeutic dose of olanzapine (20 mg/day) for 6 weeks. She has shown no response but also exhibits no side effects. The **ideal** course of action at this point would be to:

A. Obtain a plasma level of olanzapine

B. Raise the dose of olanzapine

C. Switch to a different antipsychotic

Answer to Question Thirteen

The correct answer is A.

Choice	Peer answers
Obtain a plasma level of olanzapine	71%
Raise the dose of olanzapine	15%
Switch to a different antipsychotic	14%

A – Correct. Obtaining antipsychotic plasma levels in patients who have had poor response despite a trial with an adequate dose/duration of medication can be helpful in order to rule out poor adherence, identify rapid elimination, or confirm true treatment resistance. Although not all antipsychotics have well-established therapeutic plasma levels, olanzapine is among those agents that do.

B – Incorrect. Although raising the dose of olanzapine in a patient who has neither a response nor side effects could be attempted, plasma levels – not dose – are the best guide to the extent of patient medication exposure and are the best predictors of antipsychotic response. Thus, given that the olanzapine dose is at the top of the typically recommended range, one would ideally obtain plasma levels prior to any treatment adjustment.

C – Incorrect. Given that the patient has neither a response nor any side effects, it is reasonable that her medication exposure is subtherapeutic despite being dosed in the therapeutic range. Thus, it would make sense to obtain antipsychotic plasma levels prior to switching medications.

QUESTION FOURTEEN

A 38-year-old man was diagnosed with schizophrenia 14 years ago, and over the course of his illness has taken several different antipsychotics, all with partial response and no severe side effects. He now presents with acute exacerbation of hallucinations and delusions. He recently had bowel resection due to a gastrointestinal disorder, and blood levels reveal that he is not absorbing his medications well. One option for this patient would be to prescribe heroic oral doses of his antipsychotic. Aside from this approach, which of the following antipsychotics have formulations that may be good long-term options for bypassing his problem with absorption?

A. Asenapine, paliperidone, risperidone

B. Paliperidone, risperidone, quetiapine

C. Risperidone, quetiapine, ziprasidone

D. Quetiapine, ziprasidone, asenapine

Answer to Question Fourteen

The correct answer is A.

Choice	Peer answers
Asenapine, paliperidone, risperidone	77%
Paliperidone, risperidone, quetiapine	11%
Risperidone, quetiapine, ziprasidone	7%
Quetiapine, ziprasidone, asenapine	5%

A – Correct (asenapine, paliperidone, risperidone). For patients with difficulty absorbing medications, the best options in order to reach therapeutic blood levels would be to prescribe heroic oral doses or to use parental, sublingual, or suppository administration. Asenapine has a sublingual formulation, while several atypical antipsychotics are available as long-acting injectable antipsychotics (LAI): risperidone microspheres (2-week formulation), paliperidone palmitate (4- and 12-week formulations), olanzapine pamoate (4-week formulation), aripiprazole monohydrate (4-week formulation), and aripiprazole lauroxil (4-, 6-, and 8-week formulations). Additional antipsychotics with LAI formulations include fluphenazine, haloperidol, flupenthixol, pipothiazine, and zuclopenthixol. Clozapine, olanzapine, and risperidone have orally disintegrating tablets; however, these medications are not absorbed sublingually and must be swallowed in order to undergo absorption in the gut. Chlorpromazine has a suppository formulation, and other antipsychotics may also be able to be administered as suppositories.

B – Incorrect (paliperidone, risperidone, quetiapine). Paliperidone and risperidone are both viable options, but quetiapine is only available as an oral tablet.

C – Incorrect (risperidone, quetiapine, ziprasidone). Risperidone is a viable option. However, quetiapine is only available as an oral tablet. Ziprasidone is available in an intramuscular formulation, which would bypass absorption issues, but it is for acute agitation and is not to be administered long term.

D – Incorrect (quetiapine, ziprasidone, asenapine). Asenapine is a viable option, but neither quetiapine nor ziprasidone would be (see above for explanation).

References

Stahl SM. *Case studies: Stahl's essential psychopharmacology*. New York, NY: Cambridge University Press; 2011.

Stahl SM. *Stahl's essential psychopharmacology*, fourth edition. New York, NY: Cambridge University Press; 2013. (Chapter 5)

Stahl SM. *Essential psychopharmacology, the prescriber's guide*, sixth edition. New York, NY: Cambridge University Press; 2017.

Stahl SM, **Mignon L**. *Stahl's illustrated antipsychotics*, second edition. Carlsbad, CA: NEI Press; 2009. (Chapter 5)

Psychosis and Schizophrenia and Antipsychotics

QUESTION FIFTEEN

A 28-year-old man was recently diagnosed with schizophrenia. He has a body mass index of 30, fasting triglycerides of 220 mg/dl, and fasting glucose of 114 mg/dl. Which of the following is least likely to worsen his metabolic profile?

A. Olanzapine

B. Quetiapine

C. Risperidone

D. Ziprasidone

Answer to Question Fifteen

The correct answer is D.

Choice	Peer answers
Olanzapine	13%
Quetiapine	3%
Risperidone	5%
Ziprasidone	79%

A – Incorrect. Olanzapine is one of the antipsychotics most associated with weight gain and metabolic risk and would not be a first-line option for patients who have a primary concern about metabolic issues. Clozapine also can cause problematic weight and metabolic side effects.

B – Incorrect. Quetiapine can lead to weight gain and increased triglyceride levels and may be a second-line option if a primary concern is metabolic issues.

C – Incorrect. Risperidone can lead to weight gain and increased triglyceride levels and may be a second-line option if a primary concern is metabolic issues. Paliperidone, which is the active metabolite of risperidone, can also lead to weight gain and metabolic changes. Iloperidone, asenapine, cariprazine, and brexpiprazole may also cause weight gain.

D – Correct. Ziprasidone in general seems to be weight-neutral and has been shown to lower triglyceride levels. It is therefore a recommended choice for individuals for whom metabolic issues are a primary concern. Other newer antipsychotics that may be less likely to cause weight gain or metabolic side effects include aripiprazole (although data suggest that weight gain may occur more in children and adolescents) and lurasidone.

References

Stahl SM. *Stahl's essential psychopharmacology*, fourth edition. New York, NY: Cambridge University Press; 2013. (Chapter 5)

Stahl SM. *Essential psychopharmacology, the prescriber's guide*, sixth edition. New York, NY: Cambridge University Press; 2017.

QUESTION SIXTEEN

A 27-year-old male has a history of non-adherence to oral antipsychotics, but adamantly refuses to take a long-acting injectable antipsychotic. In order to reduce his risk of relapse, which of the following oral medications might be the best choice for this patient?

A. Cariprazine

B. Clozapine

C. Perphenazine

D. Quetiapine

Answer to Question Sixteen

The correct answer is A.

Choice	Peer answers
Cariprazine	56%
Clozapine	23%
Perphenazine	9%
Quetiapine	11%

A – Correct. Cariprazine has a very long half-life: the half-life of the parent drug is 2–4 days, while the half-life of the active metabolite (didesmethyl cariprazine) is 1–3 weeks. Long half-lives mean that it will take longer to reach steady state, which can cause side effects to manifest late following treatment initiation; in addition, changes in efficacy or side effects related to dose adjustment can take longer to manifest. Long half-lives can also mean that a few missed doses may not be as detrimental in terms of risk of relapse, because residual dose can remain for several days (weeks in some cases).

B – Incorrect. Compared to other antipsychotics, clozapine has a relatively short half-life (5–16 hours); in addition, the monitoring schedule associated with clozapine may be problematic for a patient who is non-adherent to treatment.

C – Incorrect. Perphenazine has a half-life of 9.5 hours.

D – Incorrect. Quetiapine has a half-life of 6–7 hours.

References

Durgam S, Earley W, Li R et al. Long-term cariprazine treatment for the prevention of relapse in patients with schizophrenia: a randomized, double-blind, placebo-controlled trial. *Schiz Res* 2016;176:264–71.

Stahl SM. *Essential psychopharmacology, the prescriber's guide*, sixth edition. New York, NY: Cambridge University Press; 2017.

QUESTION SEVENTEEN

Carol is a 47-year-old patient with schizophrenia. She was taking a conventional antipsychotic but decided to stop taking it when she developed parkinsonian symptoms. Secondary to stopping her conventional antipsychotic, Carol's auditory hallucinations and paranoia returned, and she was rehospitalized. You recommend that she be started on an atypical antipsychotic. Which of the following has the lowest risk of extrapyramidal symptoms associated with it?

A. Asenapine

B. Iloperidone

C. Olanzapine

D. Paliperidone

Answer to Question Seventeen

The correct answer is B.

Choice	Peer answers
Asenapine	22%
Iloperidone	41%
Olanzapine	28%
Paliperidone	9%

As a class, atypical antipsychotics tend to have a decreased risk of movement disorders relative to conventional antipsychotics; however, the risk differs with each individual agent.

A – Incorrect (asenapine).

B – Correct. Of the agents listed here, iloperidone has a relatively lower risk of extrapyramidal side effects (EPS). Other agents with a relatively lower risk of EPS include clozapine and quetiapine.

C – Incorrect (olanzapine).

D – Incorrect (paliperidone).

References

Roth BL. Ki determinations, receptor binding profiles, agonist and/or antagonist functional data, HERG data, MDR1 data, etc. as appropriate was generously provided by the National Institute of Mental Health's Psychoactive Drug Screening Program, Contract # HHSN-271–2008-00025-C (NIMH PDSP). The NIMH PDSP is directed by Bryan L. Roth MD, PhD at the University of North Carolina at Chapel Hill and Project Officer Jamie Driscol at NIMH, Bethesda MD, USA. For experimental details please refer to the PDSP website http://pdsp.med.unc.edu.

Santana N, Mengod G, Artigas F. Expression of alpha 1-adrenergic receptors in rat prefrontal cortex: cellular co-localization with 5-HT2A receptors. *Int J Neuropsychopharmacol* 2013;16(5):1139–51.

Stahl SM. *Stahl's essential psychopharmacology*, fourth edition. New York, NY: Cambridge University Press; 2013.

QUESTION EIGHTEEN

Ryan is a 26-year-old white male with treatment-resistant schizo-affective disorder, depressive type, and frequent suicidal ideation and behavior. After adequate but unsuccessful trials with several mood stabilizers and atypical antipsychotics (both as monotherapy and in various combinations), you are considering a trial of clozapine. Which of the following testing should you order prior to initiating clozapine?

A. White blood cell count (WBC)

B. Absolute neutrophil count (ANC)

C. A and B

D. Neither A nor B

Answer to Question Eighteen

The correct answer is B.

Choice	Peer answers
White blood cell count (WBC)	4%
Absolute neutrophil count (ANC)	35%
A and B	61%
Neither A nor B	0%

A – Incorrect. Total white blood cell count (WBC) is no longer used when deciding whether to initiate or continue clozapine.

B – Correct. Before initiating clozapine treatment, it is necessary to obtain absolute neutrophil count (ANC). The lower ANC threshold for starting clozapine is at least 1500/μl in the general population and at least 1000/μl in individuals with benign ethnic neutropenia (BEN). BEN is a condition observed in certain ethnic groups (most commonly those of African descent, some Middle Eastern ethnic groups, and other non-Caucasian ethnic groups with darker skin). Patients with BEN have normal hematopoietic stem cell numbers and myeloid maturation, are healthy, do not suffer from repeated or severe infections, and are not at an increased risk for developing clozapine-induced neutropenia.

C – Incorrect. ANC, but not WBC, is required prior to initiating clozapine.

D – Incorrect. ANC is required prior to initiating clozapine.

References

Neuroscience Education Institute. Recommended ANC monitoring [pdf]. 2017.

Stahl SM. *Essential psychopharmacology, the prescriber's guide*, sixth edition. New York, NY: Cambridge University Press; 2017.

QUESTION NINETEEN

A 38-year-old woman was diagnosed with schizophrenia approximately 2 years ago and after multiple trials of atypical and typical antipsychotic medications she has been maintained on haloperidol for the last several months with good response. Two weeks ago she began exhibiting mild motor symptoms of parkinsonism. Which of the following would be the most appropriate adjunct medication for this patient?

A. Alpha 1 adrenergic agonist

B. Cholinesterase inhibitor

C. Histamine 1 antagonist

D. Muscarinic 1 antagonist

Answer to Question Nineteen

The correct answer is D.

Choice	Peer answers
Alpha 1 adrenergic agonist	13%
Cholinesterase inhibitor	22%
Histamine 1 antagonist	9%
Muscarinic 1 antagonist	56%

Extrapyramidal side effects (EPS) such as parkinsonism are associated with a relative deficiency of dopamine and an excess of acetylcholine in the nigrostriatal pathway. Dopamine normally suppresses acetylcholine activity; thus, blockade of dopamine 2 receptors by antipsychotics enhances release of acetylcholine and can lead to the production of parkinsonian symptoms. Increasing availability of dopamine and/or decreasing acetylcholine would therefore be expected to relieve EPS.

A – Incorrect. Haloperidol is an antagonist at the alpha 1 adrenergic receptor and an agonist would therefore reverse its effects; however, alpha 1 stimulation may actually decrease striatal dopamine release and thus would not relieve parkinsonism.

B – Incorrect. A cholinesterase inhibitor would reduce metabolism of acetylcholine and cause a further increase, rather than decrease, in this neurotransmitter.

C – Incorrect. Similarly, the histamine system is not associated with development of or relief from EPS. Some antihistamines are muscarinic 1 antagonists but their H1 antagonist properties do not regulate EPS.

D – Correct. Antagonism of the muscarinic 1 receptor for acetylcholine would prevent it from binding there and thus reduce its effects, potentially relieving EPS.

References

Stahl SM. *Stahl's essential psychopharmacology*, fourth edition. New York, NY: Cambridge University Press; 2013. (Chapter 5)

Stahl SM. *Essential psychopharmacology, the prescriber's guide*, sixth edition. New York, NY: Cambridge University Press; 2017.

Stahl SM, Mignon L. *Stahl's illustrated antipsychotics*, second edition. Carlsbad, CA: NEI Press; 2009. (Chapter 3)

QUESTION TWENTY

A 27-year-old male who has been treated with risperidone for the last 8 weeks is now having his medication changed to quetiapine. What is the recommended switching method in this situation, assuming the need to do this expeditiously, but not urgently, as an outpatient?

A. Maintain therapeutic dose of risperidone while uptitrating quetiapine to effective dose, then discontinue risperidone

B. Downtitrate risperidone over several weeks while uptitrating quetiapine over the same time period

C. Downtitrate risperidone over at least 1 week while uptitrating quetiapine over at least 2 weeks

D. Downtitrate risperidone over at least 2 weeks while uptitrating quetiapine over 1 week

Answer to Question Twenty

The correct answer is C.

Choice	Peer answers
Maintain therapeutic dose of risperidone while uptitrating quetiapine to effective dose, then discontinue risperidone	7%
Downtitrate risperidone over several weeks while uptitrating quetiapine over the same time period	24%
Downtitrate risperidone over at least 1 week while uptitrating quetiapine over at least 2 weeks	48%
Downtitrate risperidone over at least 2 weeks while uptitrating quetiapine over 1 week	21%

A – Incorrect. Maintain therapeutic dose of risperidone while uptitrating quetiapine to an effective dose, then discontinue risperidone: It is not generally recommended to maintain full therapeutic dose of one antipsychotic while uptitrating another as this can cause increased risk of side effects.

B – Incorrect. Downtitrate risperidone over several weeks while uptitrating quetiapine over the same time period: In general cross-titration with risperidone and quetiapine would not have to be this slow.

C – Correct. Downtitrate risperidone over at least 1 week while uptitrating quetiapine over at least 2 weeks: Tolerability may be best if quetiapine can be titrated up over the course of 2 weeks, while keeping the estimated D2 receptor occupancy constant as the risperidone is stopped.

D – Incorrect. Downtitrate risperidone over at least 2 weeks while uptitrating quetiapine over 1 week: Risperidone can be downtitrated faster than this. In addition, tolerability may be best if uptitration of quetiapine is slower.

References
Stahl SM. *Stahl's essential psychopharmacology*, fourth edition. New York, NY: Cambridge University Press; 2013. (Chapter 5)

Stahl SM. *Essential psychopharmacology, the prescriber's guide*, sixth edition. New York, NY: Cambridge University Press; 2017.

QUESTION TWENTY ONE

Reggie is a 30-year-old male patient with schizophrenia. He is currently taking iloperidone 24 mg/day as well as aripiprazole 15 mg/day but continues to experience visual hallucinations. To improve this patient's psychosis, it is likely necessary to further increase the blockade of dopamine D2 receptors. Which treatment strategy is likely the best course of action?

A. Increase iloperidone dose while keeping aripiprazole dose the same

B. Increase iloperidone and aripiprazole doses

C. Increase aripiprazole dose while keeping iloperidone dose the same

D. Maintain iloperidone dose and discontinue aripiprazole

Answer to Question Twenty One

The correct answer is D.

Choice	Peer answers
Increase iloperidone dose while keeping aripiprazole dose the same	33%
Increase iloperidone and aripiprazole doses	0%
Increase aripiprazole dose while keeping iloperidone dose the same	25%
Maintain iloperidone dose and discontinue aripiprazole	42%

Aripiprazole is a dopamine D2 partial agonist and is also one of the most potent agents that bind to D2 receptors. Thus, when given concomitantly with a D2 antagonist, such as iloperidone, it can actually reduce the level of D2 blockade compared to D2 antagonist monotherapy, thus reducing the antipsychotic efficacy.

A – Incorrect. Increasing the dose of iloperidone while maintaining the aripiprazole dose would not likely lead to a relevant increase in D2 blockade (and corresponding improvement of psychotic symptoms), because aripiprazole has higher affinity for the D2 receptor.

B – Incorrect. Increasing doses of both iloperidone and aripiprazole would not likely lead to improvement of psychotic symptoms, because aripiprazole would continue to compete with iloperidone at the D2 receptor.

C – Incorrect. Increasing the dose of aripiprazole may actually decrease D2 blockade rather than increase it, because aripiprazole has higher affinity for the D2 receptor than iloperidone.

D – Correct. Because aripiprazole may be reducing the level of D2 blockade relative to iloperidone monotherapy, the best strategy for increasing D2 blockade (and correspondingly improving psychotic symptoms) may be to use monotherapy.

References

Stahl SM. *Stahl's essential psychopharmacology*, fourth edition. New York, NY: Cambridge University Press; 2013.

QUESTION TWENTY TWO

A 20-year-old woman is brought in by her mother, who is concerned because in the last year her daughter has exhibited notable changes in her behavior, including deterioration in her verbal and written communication, disorganization, confusion, and poor grooming. After full assessment, you are concerned that the patient is at ultra-high risk of developing psychosis. Which of the following are approved to treat the prodromal phase of schizophrenia?

A. Aripiprazole

B. Olanzapine

C. Risperidone

D. B and C

E. No agents are approved for this use

Answer to Question Twenty Two

The correct answer is E.

Choice	Peer answers
Aripiprazole	7%
Olanzapine	0%
Risperidone	2%
B and C	13%
No agents are approved for this use	78%

A, B, C, and D – Incorrect.

E – Correct. No agents are approved for the prodromal phase of schizophrenia.

Prodrome refers to an early set of symptoms, and in schizophrenia has been characterized as the period of decreased functioning that precedes the onset of psychotic symptoms. It is not possible to predict with great accuracy who will get schizophrenia, but certain symptoms such as social withdrawal and cognitive decline can identify teenagers and young adults at high risk. A recent meta-analysis suggests that the transition to psychosis in patients at ultra-high risk is most likely to occur within the first 2 years, with half of patients who progress doing so within the first 8 months. **No drug is approved** for the social withdrawal and cognitive decline in the schizophrenia prodrome, or for the prevention of psychosis onset. Numerous studies of antipsychotics, antidepressants, and anxiolytics suggest that some patients can attain symptomatic relief and may even delay the onset of first-episode psychosis, but there is little evidence of disease modification by these medications such that schizophrenia can be prevented. Clinicians must decide whether to err on the side of undertreatment (error of omission) or on the side of overtreatment (error of commission), because prodromal cases have unpredictable outcomes.

References

Addington J, Liu L, Buchy L et al. North American Prodrome Longitudinal Study (NAPLS 2): the prodromal symptoms. *J Nerv Ment Dis* 2015;203(5):328–35.

deKoning MB, Bloemen OJN, va Amelsvoort TAMH et al. Early intervention in patients at ultra high risk of psychosis: benefits and risks. *Acta Psychiatr Scand* 2009;119:26–42.

Kempton MJ, Bonoldi I, Valmaggia L, Mcguire P, Fusar-Poli P. Speed of psychosis progression in people at ultra-high clinical risk. *JAMA Psychiatry* 2015;72(6):622–63.

McGlashan TH, Zipursky RB, Perkins D et al. Randomized, double-blind trial of olanzapine versus placebo in patients prodromally symptomatic for psychosis. *Am J Psychiatry* 2006;163:790–9.

McGorry PD, Nelson B, Amminger GP et al. Intervention in individuals at ultra high risk for psychosis: a review and future directions. *J Clin Psychiatry* 2009;70:1206–12.

Schmidt SJ, Schultze-Lutter F, Schimmelmann BG, et al. EPA guidance on the early intervention in clinical high risk states of psychoses. *Eur Psychiatry* 2015;30:388–404.

Psychosis and Schizophrenia and Antipsychotics

QUESTION TWENTY THREE

A 37-year-old woman with schizophrenia has failed to respond to two sequential adequate trials of antipsychotic monotherapy (first olanzapine, then aripiprazole). Which of the following are evidence-based treatment strategies for a patient in this situation?

A. High dose of her current monotherapy (aripiprazole)

B. Augmentation of her current monotherapy with another atypical antipsychotic

C. Switch to clozapine

D. A and C

E. A, B, and C

Psychosis and Schizophrenia and Antipsychotics

Answer to Question Twenty Three

The correct answer is C.

Choice	Peer answers
High dose of her current monotherapy (aripiprazole)	2%
Augmentation of her current monotherapy with another atypical antipsychotic	8%
Switch to clozapine	71%
A and C	5%
A, B, and C	13%

A – Incorrect. Controlled studies for high doses of antipsychotics are quite limited. In particular, the limited data that exist for aripiprazole suggest that it is not usually more effective at doses above the usual recommended range (i.e., 15–30 mg/day for psychosis). Before resorting to high-dose monotherapy, evidence-based strategies for treatment resistance should be exhausted, including the use of clozapine.

B – Incorrect. There is limited evidence to support the superior efficacy of combining antipsychotics vs. switching to clozapine or another monotherapy. Controlled studies are limited and review of the evidence that does exist (clinical trials and case reports) has not led to recommendations for antipsychotic polypharmacy in routine clinical practice.

C – Correct. After failure of two sequential adequate trials of antipsychotic monotherapy, the recommended and evidence-based treatment strategy is to switch to clozapine.

D – Incorrect (A and C).

E – Incorrect (A, B, and C).

References

Pandurangi AK, Dalkilic A. Polypharmacy with second-generation antipsychotics: a review of evidence. *J Psychiatr Pract* 2008;14:345.

Royal College of Psychiatrists. CR138. Consensus Statement on High-Dose Antipsychotic Medication. 2006. www.rcpsych.ac.uk/files/pdfversion/CR138.pdf.

Stahl SM. *Essential psychopharmacology, the prescriber's guide*, sixth edition. New York, NY: Cambridge University Press; 2017.

QUESTION TWENTY FOUR

A 16-year-old female is brought to the hospital by her mother because she is complaining that her neighbors spy on her and submit their observations to the government. After evaluation, she is diagnosed with schizophrenia and prescribed risperidone. Which of the following is the appropriate target therapeutic dose for this patient?

A. 0.5 mg/day

B. 3 mg/day

C. 6 mg/day

D. 12 mg/day

Answer to Question Twenty Four

The correct answer is B.

Choice	Peer answers
0.5 mg/day	7%
3 mg/day	71%
6 mg/day	21%
12 mg/day	1%

A – Incorrect. 0.5 mg/day: Although this is the recommended starting dose for adolescents with schizophrenia (ages 13–17), the recommended therapeutic dose is higher.

B – Correct. 3 mg/day: This is the recommended therapeutic dose for adolescents (ages 13–17) with schizophrenia.

C – Incorrect. 6 mg/day: This is within the recommended dose range for adults with schizophrenia; however, in studies of adolescents doses above 3 mg/day were associated with additional side effects and no additional efficacy.

D – Incorrect. 12 mg/day: Doses above 6 mg/day have not been studied in adolescents with schizophrenia.

References

Stahl SM. *Stahl's essential psychopharmacology*, fourth edition. New York, NY: Cambridge University Press; 2013. (Chapter 5)

Stahl SM. *Essential psychopharmacology, the prescriber's guide*, sixth edition. New York, NY: Cambridge University Press; 2017.

CHAPTER PEER COMPARISON

For the Psychosis and Schizophrenia section, the correct answer was selected 62% of the time.

3 UNIPOLAR DEPRESSION AND ANTIDEPRESSANTS

QUESTION ONE

A 26-year-old woman began treatment for a major depressive episode 8 months ago. Two months into her treatment she began to experience noticeable symptom improvement, and for the last 5 months she has been nearly symptom-free. According to the general consensus, her current state could be classified as a:

A. Response

B. Remission

C. Recovery

D. Relapse

E. Recurrence

Answer to Question One

The correct answer is B.

Choice	Peer answers
Response	15%
Remission	76%
Recovery	9%
Relapse	0%
Recurrence	0%

A – Incorrect. A response is characterized as at least a 50% improvement of symptoms, whereas this patient has experienced a near elimination of symptoms.

B – Correct. When treatment of depression results in removal of essentially all symptoms, as with this patient, it is called remission for the first several months (e.g., up to 6 months).

C – Incorrect. Recovery is described as being symptom-free for 6 months or more.

D – Incorrect. When depression returns before there is a full remission of symptoms or within the first several months following remission of symptoms, it is called a relapse.

E – Incorrect. When depression symptoms return after a patient has recovered, it is called a recurrence.

References

Stahl SM. *Stahl's essential psychopharmacology*, fourth edition. New York, NY: Cambridge University Press; 2013. (Chapter 7)

Zimmerman M, McGlinchey JB, Posternak MA, Friedman M, Attiullah N, Boerescu D. How should remission from depression be defined? The depressed patient's perspective. *Am J Psychiatry* 2006;163: 148–50.

QUESTION TWO

A 38-year-old patient with depression presents with depressed mood, anhedonia, and loss of energy. These symptoms can be conceptualized as reflecting reduced positive affect; such a categorization is theoretically useful because it may direct treatment choice. Specifically, symptoms of reduced positive affect are hypothetically more likely to respond to agents that enhance:

A. Serotonin and possibly dopamine function

B. Dopamine and possibly norepinephrine function

C. Norepinephrine and possibly serotonin function

Unipolar Depression and Antidepressants

Answer to Question Two

The correct answer is B.

Choice	Peer answers
Serotonin and possibly dopamine function	31%
Dopamine and possibly norepinephrine function	57%
Norepinephrine and possibly serotonin function	13%

Mood-related symptoms of depression can be characterized by their affective expression – that is, whether they cause a reduction in positive affect (e.g., depressed mood, anhedonia) or an increase in negative affect (e.g., anxiety, irritability). This concept is based on the fact that there are diffuse anatomic connections of monoamines throughout the brain, with diffuse dopamine dysfunction in this system driving predominantly the reduction of positive affect, diffuse serotonin dysfunction driving predominantly the increase in negative affect, and norepinephrine dysfunction being involved in both.

A – Incorrect. Although dopaminergic dysfunction is thought to be related to decreased positive affect, serotonergic dysfunction is thought to be related to increased negative affect.

B – Correct. Because reduced positive affect is thought to be related to dopamine dysfunction and possibly norepinephrine dysfunction, enhancing one or both of these neurotransmitters would theoretically be most likely to improve these symptoms.

C – Incorrect. Although norepinephrine dysfunction is thought to be involved in reduced positive affect, serotonergic dysfunction is thought to be related to increased negative affect.

References
Stahl SM. *Stahl's essential psychopharmacology*, fourth edition. New York, NY: Cambridge University Press; 2013. (Chapter 7)

Unipolar Depression and Antidepressants

QUESTION THREE

A 36-year-old man with major depressive disorder is having lab work done to assess his levels of inflammatory markers. Based on the current evidence regarding inflammation in depression, which of the following results would you most likely suspect for this patient?

A. Elevated levels of tumor necrosis factor–alpha (TNF-alpha)

B. Reduced levels of interleukin 6 (IL-6)

C. Both A and B

D. Neither A nor B

Answer to Question Three

The correct answer is A.

Choice	Peer answers
Elevated levels of tumor necrosis factor-alpha (TNF-alpha)	45%
Reduced levels of interleukin 6 (IL-6)	9%
Both A and B	33%
Neither A nor B	12%

A – Correct. There is growing evidence that inflammation may play an important role in the pathophysiology of major depression. Clinical studies have shown that depressed patients have significantly higher concentrations of several inflammatory markers, including the pro-inflammatory cytokines TNF-alpha, interleukin 6, and interleukin 1. Patients with depression also have higher concentrations of C-reactive protein, which is synthesized by the liver in response to pro-inflammatory cytokines. Furthermore, both cytokines and cytokine inducers can cause symptoms of depression. For example, as many as 50% of patients receiving chronic therapy with the cytokine interferon develop symptoms consistent with idiopathic depression.

B, C, and D – Incorrect.

References

Bhattacharya A, Derecki NC, Lovenberg TW, Drevets WC. Role of neuro-immunological factors in the pathophysiology of mood disorders. *Psychopharmacology (Berl)* 2016;233(9):1623–36.

Dowlati Y, Herrmann N, Swardfager JW, et al. A meta-analysis of cytokines in major depression. *Biol Psychiatry* 2010;67:446–57.

Haroon E, Raison CL, Miller AH. Psychoneuroimmunology meets neuropsychopharmacology: translational implications of the impact of inflammation on behavior. *Neuropsychopharmacology* 2012;37:137–62.

Howren MB, Lamkin DM, Suls J. Associations of depression with C-reactive protein, IL-1, and IL-6: a meta-analysis. *Psychosom Med* 2009;71:171–86.

Raison CL, Miller AH. Is depression an inflammatory disorder? *Curr Psychiatry Rep* 2011;13:467–75.

QUESTION FOUR

Denise is a 56–year–old perimenopausal patient with a history of depression. Her depressed mood seems to be responding to her current treatment with the selective serotonin reuptake inhibitor (SSRI) fluoxetine (40 mg/day); however, she is troubled by hot flashes and night sweats, and she reports some residual depressed mood. Which treatment strategy is likely to optimize this patient's chance for remission?

A. Maintain current fluoxetine dose

B. Decrease fluoxetine dose

C. Switch to a different selective serotonin reuptake inhibitor (SSRI)

D. Switch to a serotonin and norepinephrine reuptake inhibitor (SNRI)

Answer to Question Four

The correct answer is D.

Choice	Peer answers
Maintain current fluoxetine dose	9%
Decrease fluoxetine dose	8%
Switch to a different selective serotonin reuptake inhibitor (SSRI)	13%
Switch to a serotonin and norepinephrine reuptake inhibitor (SNRI)	70%

A – Incorrect. The ultimate goal of depression treatment should be the amelioration of all symptoms rather than improvement in depressive symptoms alone. Residual symptoms are often predictive of poor long-term outcomes, including increased disability, more frequent relapses, relationship and work difficulties, and suicide. Although this patient is responding to her current treatment with fluoxetine, she is experiencing residual depressed mood and vasomotor symptoms. The presence of vasomotor symptoms indicates that this patient's estrogen levels are in flux, putting her at risk for depressive relapse. In order to prevent relapse and achieve remission, a change in treatment strategy is warranted.

B – Incorrect. This patient is having at least partial response to her current dose of fluoxetine. Decreasing the dose is likely to diminish the therapeutic effects of fluoxetine and not improve her vasomotor symptoms.

C – Incorrect. Vasomotor symptoms are thought to be due to dysfunction in both serotonin and norepinephrine neurotransmission, specifically in the hypothalamus. Although SSRIs may have some efficacy in the treatment of both depression and vasomotor symptoms, SNRIs have been shown to be more effective and are the treatment of choice for patients with these symptoms.

D – Correct. Vasomotor symptoms, including hot flashes and night sweats, are associated with estrogen fluctuations, such as those that occur during the perimenopausal period of the female lifespan. Estrogen fluctuations lead to dysregulation of the serotonergic and noradrenergic systems that are thought to mediate both vasomotor symptoms and depression. Vasomotor symptoms may signal vulnerability to the onset or recurrence of a major depressive episode; this is not surprising because the presence of vasomotor symptoms indicates that estrogen is in flux even if depressive symptoms are responding to antidepressant treatment. Although SSRIs may have some efficacy in the treatment of both depression and vasomotor symptoms, SNRIs have been shown to be more effective and are the treatment of choice for patients with these symptoms.

References

Stahl SM. Vasomotor symptoms and depression in women, part 1: role of vasomotor symptoms in signaling the onset or relapse of a major depressive episode. *J Clin Psychiatry* 2009;70(1):11–2.

Stahl SM. Vasomotor symptoms and depression in women, part 2: treatments that cause remission and prevent relapses of major depressive episodes overlap with treatments for vasomotor symptoms. *J Clin Psychiatry* 2009;70(3):310–1.

QUESTION FIVE

Margaret is a 42-year-old patient with untreated depression. She is reluctant to begin antidepressant treatment due to concerns about treatment-induced weight gain. Which of the following antidepressant treatments is associated with the greatest risk of weight gain?

A. Escitalopram

B. Fluoxetine

C. Mirtazapine

D. Vilazodone

Answer to Question Five

The correct answer is C.

Choice	Peer answers
Escitalopram	0%
Fluoxetine	3%
Mirtazapine	95%
Vilazodone	1%

A – Incorrect. Although weight gain may occur, it is not commonly reported with escitalopram, and a meta-analysis suggests that the risk of both short- and long-term weight gain with escitalopram is low.

B – Incorrect. Although weight gain may occur, it is not commonly reported with fluoxetine and a meta-analysis did not find significant increase in weight over the short or long term. Some patients actually experience short-term weight loss with fluoxetine.

C – Correct. Meta-analysis has shown that mirtazapine, an alpha 2 antagonist, may cause both short- and long-term weight gain. This is consistent with its secondary pharmacologic properties: mirtazapine is an antagonist at both serotonin 2C and histamine 1 receptors, the combination of which has been proposed to cause weight gain. However, it should be noted that average weight gain with any antidepressant is small, and rather than a widespread effect it may instead be that a small number of individuals experience significant weight gain due to their genetic predispositions and other factors.

D – Incorrect. Although weight gain may occur, studies with vilazodone have suggested a lower risk for weight gain compared to many other antidepressants that block serotonin reuptake; however, head-to-head studies have not been conducted.

References
Serretti A, Mandelli L. Antidepressants and body weight: a comprehensive review and meta-analysis. *J Clin Psychiatry* 2010;71(10): 1259–72.

Stahl SM. *Stahl's essential psychopharmacology, the prescriber's guide*, sixth edition. New York, NY: Cambridge University Press; 2017.

QUESTION SIX

A 52-year-old man presents to the emergency room with symptoms of hypertensive crisis after an evening dining out with friends. He is currently taking a monoamine oxidase inhibitor (MAOI). Which of the following foods must be avoided by patients taking MAOIs?

A. Fresh fish

B. Aged cheese

C. Bananas

D. Bottled beer

E. All of these must be avoided

F. None of these must be avoided

Answer to Question Six

The correct answer is B.

Choice	Peer answers
Fresh fish	0%
Aged cheese	75%
Bananas	0%
Bottled beer	1%
All of these must be avoided	22%
None of these must be avoided	2%

Tyramine content in food can instigate a hypertensive crisis in patients taking MAOIs. Meals considered to contain a high level of tyramine content generally include 40 mg of tyramine.

Foods to AVOID*	Foods ALLOWED
Dried, aged, smoked, fermented, spoiled, or improperly stored meat, poultry, and fish	Fresh or processed meat, poultry, and fish
Broad bean pods	All other vegetables
Aged cheeses	Processed cheese slices, cottage cheese, ricotta cheese, cream cheese, yogurt
Tap and unpasteurized beer	Bottled or canned beer and alcohol
Marmite	Brewer's and baker's yeast
Soy products/tofu	Peanuts
Banana peel	Bananas, avocados, raspberries
Sauerkraut, kimchee	
Tyramine-containing nutritional supplements	

*Not necessary for 6-mg transdermal or low-dose oral selegiline.

A – Incorrect. Fresh fish does not have a high tyramine content and can therefore be safely consumed when one is taking an MAOI.

B – Correct. Aged cheeses in general have high tyramine content and must be avoided when a patient is taking an MAOI.

C – Incorrect. Bananas that are not overripe do not have a high tyramine content and can therefore be safely consumed when one is taking an MAOI. However, banana peels and bananas that are overripe should be avoided.

D – Incorrect. Bottled beer does not have a high tyramine content and can therefore be safely consumed when one is taking an MAOI.

E and F – Incorrect.

References

Shulman KI, **Walker SE**. Refining the MAOI diet: tyramine content of pizzas and soy products. *J Clin Psychiatry* 1999;60(3):191–3.

Shulman KI, **Walker SE**. A reevaluation of dietary restrictions for irreversible monoamine oxidase inhibitors. *Psychiatr Ann* 2001;31(6): 378–84.

Shulman KI, **Walker SE**, **MacKenzie S**, **Knowles S**. Dietary restriction, tyramine, and the use of monoamine oxidase inhibitors. *J Clin Psychopharmacol* 1989;9(6):397–402.

QUESTION SEVEN

A 48-year-old woman with a history of treatment-resistant depression is currently taking duloxetine 60 mg/day with partial response as well as trazodone 50 mg/day for insomnia. She states that she feels empty and useless, and she admits to having thoughts of death. She states that she does not have plans to kill herself because it would harm her family and pets. Her clinician decides to try tranylcypromine, a monoamine oxidase inhibitor (MAOI) and one of the few agents that she has not yet tried. Which of the patient's current medications would you discontinue BEFORE initiating tranylcypromine?

A. Duloxetine

B. Trazodone

C. Both duloxetine and trazodone

D. Neither duloxetine nor trazodone

Answer to Question Seven

The correct answer is A.

Choice	Peer answers
Duloxetine	45%
Trazodone	6%
Both duloxetine and trazodone	47%
Neither duloxetine nor trazodone	1%

A – Correct. Duloxetine is a serotonin and norepinephrine reuptake inhibitor. Inhibition of the serotonin transporter leads to increased synaptic availability of serotonin. Similarly, inhibition of MAO leads to increased serotonin levels. In combination, these two mechanisms can cause excessive stimulation of postsynaptic serotonin receptors, which has the potential to cause a fatal "serotonin syndrome" or "serotonin toxicity." Because of the risk of serotonin toxicity, complete washout of duloxetine is necessary before starting an MAOI. Duloxetine must be downtitrated as tolerated, after which one must wait 5 half-lives of duloxetine (at least 3–4 days) before initiating the MAOI.

B – Incorrect. Although trazodone does have serotonin reuptake inhibition at antidepressant doses (150 mg or higher), this property is not clinically relevant at the low doses used for insomnia. In fact, because there is a required gap in antidepressant treatment when switching to or from an MAOI, low-dose trazodone can be useful as a bridging agent when switching.

C and D – Incorrect.

References

Dvir Y, **Smallwood P**. Serotonin syndrome: a complex but easily avoidable condition. *Gen Hosp Psychiatry* 2008;30(3):284–7.

Stahl SM. *Stahl's essential psychopharmacology*, fourth edition. New York, NY: Cambridge University Press; 2013. (Chapter 7)

Stahl SM. *Stahl's essential psychopharmacology, the prescriber's guide*, sixth edition. New York, NY: Cambridge University Press; 2017.

Wimbiscus M, **Kostenkjo O**, **Malone D**. MAO inhibitors: risks, benefits, and lore. *Cleveland Clinic J Med* 2010;77(12):859–82.

QUESTION EIGHT

A 56-year-old male patient with major depression is brought to the emergency room with cardiac arrhythmia and possible cardiac arrest. While at the hospital, he suffers a seizure. His wife states that he may have ingested an increased dose of his medication. Which of the following is most likely responsible for this apparent overdose reaction?

A. Clomipramine

B. Atomoxetine

C. Fluvoxamine

D. Venlafaxine

Answer to Question Eight

The correct answer is A.

Choice	Peer answers
Clomipramine	83%
Atomoxetine	5%
Fluvoxamine	3%
Venlafaxine	9%

A – Correct. Clomipramine, a tricyclic antidepressant (TCA), may be most likely to cause these effects in overdose. TCAs block voltage-sensitive sodium channels (VSSCs) in both the brain and the heart. This action is weak at therapeutic doses, but in overdose may lead to coma, seizures, and cardiac arrhythmia, and may even prove fatal.

B – Incorrect. Atomoxetine, a norepinephrine reuptake inhibitor, does not block VSSCs and is not noted to have severe cardiac impairments upon overdose; rather, sedation, agitation, hyperactivity, abnormal behavior and GI symptoms are most commonly reported.

C – Incorrect. Fluvoxamine, a selective serotonin reuptake inhibitor (SSRI), also does not block VSSCs and does not generally cause severe cardiac impairment in overdose.

D – Incorrect. Venlafaxine is a serotonin and norepinephrine reuptake inhibitor (SNRI). Although some data have suggested that SNRIs can affect heart function in overdose and also may carry increased risk of death in overdose compared to selective serotonin reuptake inhibitors, their toxicity in overdose is less than that for tricyclic antidepressants.

References
Stahl SM. *Stahl's essential psychopharmacology*, fourth edition. New York, NY: Cambridge University Press; 2013. (Chapter 7)

Thanacoody HK, **Thomas SH**. Tricyclic antidepressant poisoning: cardiovascular toxicity. *Toxicol Rev* 2005;24(3):205–14.

QUESTION NINE

A 65-year-old patient on theophylline for chronic obstructive pulmonary disease (COPD) and fluvoxamine for recurring depressive episodes required a decreased dose of theophylline due to increased blood levels of the drug. Which of the following pharmacokinetic properties may be responsible for this?

A. Inhibition of CYP450 1A2 by fluvoxamine

B. Inhibition of CYP450 2D6 by fluvoxamine

C. Inhibition of CYP450 3A4 by fluvoxamine

Answer to Question Nine

The correct answer is A.

Choice	Peer answers
Inhibition of CYP450 1A2 by fluvoxamine	42%
Inhibition of CYP450 2D6 by fluvoxamine	37%
Inhibition of CYP450 3A4 by fluvoxamine	22%

A – Correct. Fluvoxamine is a strong inhibitor of CYP450 1A2. Theophylline is metabolized in part by CYP450 1A2, and thus strong inhibition of this enzyme by fluvoxamine may require a dose reduction of theophylline if the two are given concomitantly, so as to avoid increased blood levels of the drug.

B – Incorrect. Of all selective serotonin reuptake inhibitors (SSRIs), fluvoxamine shows the least interaction with CYP450 2D6.

C – Incorrect. Fluvoxamine is also a moderate inhibitor of CYP450 3A4, but because theophylline is neither a substrate nor an inhibitor of 3A4, this should not affect theophylline blood levels.

References

Stahl SM. *Stahl's essential psychopharmacology*, fourth edition. New York, NY: Cambridge University Press; 2013. (Chapter 7)

Stahl SM. *Stahl's essential psychopharmacology, the prescriber's guide*, sixth edition. New York, NY: Cambridge University Press; 2017.

QUESTION TEN

Mike is a 31-year-old patient with major depressive disorder (MDD) whose depression is responding well to the serotonin and norepinephrine reuptake inhibitor (SNRI) venlafaxine XR (150 mg/day). However, the patient acknowledges that he and his wife have been having relationship problems because of the patient's poor libido. The patient experienced this problem prior to being diagnosed and treated for MDD, but he has found that the venlafaxine has worsened this troubling symptom despite the fact that his mood has improved. Which of the following treatment strategies would you recommend for this patient?

A. Decrease venlafaxine dose

B. Switch to a norepinephrine and dopamine reuptake inhibitor (NDRI)

C. Switch to a selective serotonin reuptake inhibitor (SSRI)

D. Augment current venlafaxine dose with a phosphodiesterase-5 (e.g., sildenafil)

Answer to Question Ten

The correct answer is B.

Choice	Peer answers
Decrease venlafaxine dose	10%
Switch to a norepinephrine and dopamine reuptake inhibitor (NDRI)	58%
Switch to a selective serotonin reuptake inhibitor (SSRI)	1%
Augment current venlafaxine dose with a phosphodiesterase-5 (e.g., sildenafil)	32%

The prevalence of sexual dysfunction, including diminished libido, impaired arousal, and lack of orgasm, is high among patients with MDD, and sexual dysfunction may worsen with antidepressant treatment (particularly treatment with a serotonin reuptake inhibitor). Exacerbation of sexual dysfunction by antidepressant treatment is one of the most common factors reported to cause treatment non–adherence or discontinuation.

A – Incorrect. With regards to the diagnostic criteria for depression, this patient is responding well to his current dose of venlafaxine. Although lowering the dose of venlafaxine may improve this patient's sexual function, a dose reduction may also increase his risk of depressive relapse.

B – Correct. Pharmacological agents that increase dopaminergic neurotransmission and/or decrease serotonergic neurotransmission are often effective in ameliorating sexual dysfunction. Switching to (or augmenting with) an NDRI such as bupropion would be expected to increase dopaminergic neurotransmission and improve sexual function.

C – Incorrect. Of the available antidepressant treatments, SSRIs are associated with the greatest risk of worsening sexual function, so switching from venlafaxine to an SSRI would not be expected to improve sexual functioning.

D – Incorrect. Although it is usually best to try another antidepressant monotherapy before resorting to augmentation strategies for the treatment of side effects, for a patient such as this who is otherwise responding well it might be reasonable to augment. However, phosphodiesterase-5 inhibitors do not increase desire and thus would not be a good option to treat this patient's specific problems with sexual function.

References

Kennedy SH, Rizvi S. Sexual dysfunction, depression, and the impact of antidepressants. *J Clin Psychopharmacol* 2009;29(2):157–64.

Serretti A, Chiesa A. Sexual side effects of pharmacological treatment of psychiatric diseases. *Clin Pharmacol Ther* 2011;89(1):142–7.

Unipolar Depression and Antidepressants

QUESTION ELEVEN

Serotonin 3 antagonists may have clinical utility as adjuncts for the treatment of:

A. Cognitive symptoms

B. Depressed mood

C. Both of the above

D. None of the above

Answer to Question Eleven

The correct answer is C.

Choice	Peer answers
Cognitive symptoms	24%
Depressed mood	6%
Both of the above	60%
None of the above	10%

A and B – Correct. Serotonergic neurons synapse with noradrenergic neurons, cholinergic neurons, and GABAergic interneurons, all of which contain serotonin 3 receptors. When serotonin is released, it binds to serotonin 3 receptors on GABAergic neurons, which release GABA onto noradrenergic and cholinergic neurons, thus reducing release of norepinephrine and acetylcholine, respectively. In addition, serotonin may bind to serotonin 3 receptors on noradrenergic and cholinergic neurons, further reducing release of those neurotransmitters. This may theoretically contribute to symptoms of depressed mood and impaired cognition.

C – Correct. Cognitive symptoms and depressed mood are the correct answers.

D – Incorrect.

References

Artigas F. Serotonin receptors involved in antidepressant effects. *Pharmacol Ther* 2013;137:119–31.

Carr GV, Lucki I. The role of serotonin receptor subtypes in treating depression: a review of animal studies. *Psychopharmacology* 2011;213: 265–8.

Ciranna L. Serotonin as a modulator of glutamate- and GABA-mediated neurotransmission: implications in physiological functions and in pathology. *Curr Neuropharmacol* 2006;4(2):101–14.

Ohno Y, Shimizu S, Tokudome K. Pathophysiological roles of serotonergic system in regulating extrapyramidal motor functions. *Biol Pharm Bull* 2013;36(9):1396–400.

Shimizu S, Mizuguchi Y, Ohno Y. Improving the treatment of schizophrenia: role of 5HT receptors in modulating cognitive and extrapyramidal motor functions. *CNS Neurol Dis Drug Targets* 2013;12: 861–9.

Siarey RJ, **Andreasen M**, **Lambert JD**. Serotoninergic modulation of excitability in area CA1 of the *in vitro* rat hippocampus. *Neurosci Lett* 1995;199(3):211–4.

Stahl SM. *Stahl's essential psychopharmacology*, fourth edition. New York, NY: Cambridge University Press; 2013.

Zhou FM, **Hablitz JJ**. Activation of serotonin receptors modulates synaptic transmission in rat cerebral cortex. *J Neurophysiol* 1999;82(6): 2989–99.

Unipolar Depression and Antidepressants

QUESTION TWELVE

A 36-year-old patient has only partially responded to his second monotherapy with a first-line antidepressant. Which of the following has the best evidence of efficacy for augmenting antidepressants in patients with inadequate response?

A. Adding an atypical antipsychotic

B. Adding buspirone

C. Adding a stimulant

Answer to Question Twelve

The correct answer is A.

Choice	Peer answers
Adding an atypical antipsychotic	86%
Adding buspirone	11%
Adding a stimulant	3%

A – Correct. Atypical antipsychotics have been studied as adjuncts to selective serotonin reuptake inhibitors (SSRIs) and serotonin and norepinephrine reuptake inhibitors (SNRIs), with approvals for aripiprazole, brexpiprazole, quetiapine XR, and olanzapine (in combination with fluoxetine). Overall, most studies of atypical antipsychotics show a benefit of combination treatment over monotherapy, although effect sizes have been modest. Although atypical antipsychotics have the best evidence of efficacy for augmenting antidepressants in patients with inadequate response, their adverse event profiles may still put them later in the treatment algorithm.

B – Incorrect. Although adding buspirone, a serotonin 1A partial agonist, to a first-line antidepressant makes sense mechanistically, the limited data that exist are mixed/weak.

C – Incorrect. The limited controlled data for stimulant augmentation in depression show a trend of benefit; however, this strategy is not as well documented as is augmentation with atypical antipsychotics.

References

Bech P, Fava M, Trivedi MH, Wisniewski SR, Rush AJ. Outcomes on the pharmacopsychometric triangle in bupropion-SR vs. buspirone augmentation of citalopram in the STAR*D trial. *Acta Psychiatr Scand* 2012;125(4):342–8.

Citrome L. Adjunctive aripiprazole, olanzapine, or quetiapine for major depressive disorder: an analysis of number needed to treat, number needed to harm, and likelihood to be helped or harmed. *Postgrad Med* 2010;122(4):39–48.

Trivedi MH, Cutler, AJ, Richards C et al. A randomized controlled trial of the efficacy and safety of lisdexamfetamine dimesylate as augmentation therapy in adults with residual symptoms of major depressive disorder after treatment with escitalopram. *J Clin Psychiatry* 2013;74(8):802–9.

QUESTION THIRTEEN

A 44-year-old woman has been taking a selective seratonin reuptake inhibitor (SSRI) for 3 months. At her follow-up visit, she informs you that although her mood has improved with treatment, she is having problems engaging in sexual activity with her husband. What pharmacological treatment option might be appropriate to address her sexual dysfunction?

A. 5HT2 antagonist

B. 5HT3 antagonist

C. 5HT6 antagonist

Answer to Question Thirteen

The correct answer is A.

Choice	Peer answers
5HT2 antagonist	58%
5HT3 antagonist	25%
5HT6 antagonist	17%

A – Correct. Antidepressant-induced sexual dysfunction is hypothesized to be largely due to 5HT stimulation of 5HT2 receptors and the associated downstream decrease in dopamine. 5HT2 antagonist and agents that lack or counteract this property may be least likely to cause sexual dysfunction.

B – Incorrect. 5HT3 antagonist may enhance cognition, have anxiolytic properties and reduce extrapyramidal side effects (EPS).

C – Incorrect. 5HT6 antagonist may regulate the release of BDNF and regulate aspects of learning and memory.

References

Artigas F. Serotonin receptors involved in antidepressant effects. *Pharmacol Ther* 2013;137:119–31.

Morehouse R, Macqueen G, Kennedy SH. Barriers to achieving treatment goals: a focus on sleep disturbance and sexual dysfunction. *J Affect Disord* 2011;132(Suppl 1):S14–20.

Ohno Y, Shimizu S, Tokudome K. Pathophysiological roles of serotonergic system in regulating extrapyramidal motor functions. *Biol Pharm Bull* 2013;36(9):1396–400.

Shimizu S, Mizuguchi Y, Ohno Y. Improving the treatment of schizophrenia: role of 5HT receptors in modulating cognitive and extrapyramidal motor functions. *CNS Neurol Dis Drug Targets* 2013;12: 861–9.

Stahl SM. *Stahl's essential psychopharmacology*, fourth edition. New York, NY: Cambridge University Press; 2013.

QUESTION FOURTEEN

After being treated with sertraline for over a year, a 23-year-old man continues to suffer from significant symptoms of depressed mood and intermittent anxiety. He has recently been admitted to a substance dependence treatment program for alcohol use (up to 15 drinks per day for the last 2 years) and has been sober for 2 weeks. Psychotherapy within the program reveals that his depressed mood pre-dated the start of his heavy drinking. There is no current suicidal ideation and no history of attempted suicide. At this point, the patient has discontinued sertraline by choice. Is he a reasonable candidate for transcranial magnetic stimulation (TMS)?

A. No; he has only had one medication trial, and at least two failed trials are required before considering TMS

B. No; there is possible alteration of consciousness due to the need of anesthesia, which would interfere with his psychotherapy

C. No; his recent alcohol dependence is a contraindication for TMS

D. Yes; he fulfills criteria to qualify for a trial of TMS

Answer to Question Fourteen

The correct answer is D.

Choice	Peer answers
No; he has only had one medication trial, and at least two failed trials are required before considering TMS	43%
No; there is possible alteration of consciousness due to the need of anesthesia, which would interfere with his psychotherapy	1%
No; his recent alcohol dependence is a contraindication for TMS	12%
Yes; he fulfills criteria to qualify for a trial of TMS	44%

TMS involves an electromagnetic coil placed on the scalp, creating a magnetic field that penetrates the skull by a few centimeters. This depolarizes neurons in the superficial cortex; through neural pathways, this local stimulation causes functional changes in other brain regions. Its approval is based on a study of high-frequency TMS over the left dorsolateral prefrontal cortex (DLPFC); however, low-frequency right-sided stimulation has also shown efficacy.

A – Incorrect. TMS is approved for treatment-resistant depression, defined as having failed at least one (not two) pharmacological trials in the current episode.

B – Incorrect. TMS is generally done on an outpatient basis, requires no anesthesia, and does not involve loss of consciousness.

C – Incorrect. Recent alcohol dependence is not a contraindication for TMS. The only contraindication is for patients with ferromagnetic metal within 30 cm of where the electromagnetic coil is placed. Caution should be exercised for patients with an implantable device controlled by physiological signs.

D – Correct.

References

Berlim MT, **Van den Eynde F**, **Daskalakis JZ**. Clinically meaningful efficacy and acceptability of low-frequency repetitive transcranial magnetic stimulation (rTMS) for treating primary major depression: a meta-analysis of randomized, double-blind and sham-controlled trials. *Neuropsychopharmacology* 2013;38:543–51.

Blumberger DM, Mulsant BH, Daskalakis ZJ. What is the role of brain stimulation therapies in the treatment of depression? *Curr Psychiatry Rep* 2013;15(7):368.

Kalu UG, Sexton CE, Loo CK, Ebmeier KP. Transcranial direct current stimulation in the treatment of major depression: a meta-analysis. *Psychological Med* 2012;42(9):1791–800.

O'Reardon JP, Solvason HB, Janicak PG et al. Efficacy and safety of transcranial magnetic stimulation in the acute treatment of major depression: a multisite randomized controlled trial. *Biol Psychiatry* 2007;62(11):1208–16.

Unipolar Depression and Antidepressants

QUESTION FIFTEEN

A 36-year-old woman is suffering from her third major depressive episode. She has not experienced improvement despite adequate trials of several different antidepressants and is now undergoing electroconvulsive therapy (ECT). She did not respond until the ninth session, but has now shown progressive improvement following her tenth, eleventh, and twelfth sessions. What would be the recommended next step for this patient?

A. Discontinue ECT and switch to a medication treatment

B. Continue ECT until she reaches a plateau of improvement, then initiate medication treatment

C. Continue ECT indefinitely (barring any significant side effects) to prevent relapse

Answer to Question Fifteen

The correct answer is B.

Choice	Peer answers
Discontinue ECT and switch to a medication treatment	6%
Continue ECT until she reaches a plateau of improvement, then initiate medication treatment	75%
Continue ECT indefinitely (barring any significant side effects) to prevent relapse	19%

A and C – Incorrect.

B – Correct. Existing data and expert clinical opinion support the idea that ECT response can be relatively rapid, often occurring after a few sessions. Consistent with this, the acute course of ECT treatment is typically 6–12 treatments and does not generally exceed 20 treatments. However, it is important that treatment continues until symptoms remit or plateau, because relapse rates are higher if ECT is discontinued prematurely.

References

Gelenberg AJ, **Freeman MP**, **Markowitz JC** et al. *Practice guideline for the treatment of patients with major depressive disorder*, third edition. APA; 2010.

Husain MM, **Rush AJ**, **Fink M** et al. Speed of response and remission in major depressive disorder with acute electroconvulsive therapy (ECT): a Consortium for Research in ECT (CORE) report. *J Clin Psychiatry* 2004;65(4):485–91.

Marangell LB, **Martinez M**, **Jurdi RA**, **Zboyan H**. Neurostimulation therapies in depression: a review of new modalities. *Acta Psychiatr Scand* 2007;116:174–81.

QUESTION SIXTEEN

A 34-year-old man with depression characterized by depressed mood, sleep difficulties, and concentration problems has not responded well to a selective serotonin reuptake inhibitor (SSRI) or a serotonin and norepinephrine reuptake inhibitor. His clinician elects to switch him to vortioxetine, which has prominent 5HT7 antagonism. What may be a primary function of these receptors?

A. Regulation of serotonin–acetylcholine interactions

B. Regulation of serotonin–dopamine interactions

C. Regulation of serotonin–glutamate interactions

D. Regulation of serotonin–norepinephrine interactions

Unipolar Depression and Antidepressants

Answer to Question Sixteen

The correct answer is C.

Choice	Peer answers
Regulation of serotonin–acetylcholine interactions	19%
Regulation of serotonin–dopamine interactions	21%
Regulation of serotonin–glutamate interactions	46%
Regulation of serotonin–norepinephrine interactions	14%

A, B, and D – Incorrect.

C – Correct. 5HT7 receptors are postsynaptic G-protein-linked receptors. They are localized in the cortex, hippocampus, hypothalamus, thalamus, and brainstem raphe nuclei, where they regulate mood, circadian rhythms, sleep, learning, and memory. A major function of these receptors may be to regulate serotonin–glutamate interactions.

Serotonin can both activate and inhibit glutamate release from cortical pyramidal neurons. Serotonin released from neurons in the raphe nucleus can bind to 5HT2A receptors on pyramidal glutamate neurons in the prefrontal cortex, activating glutamate release. However, serotonin also binds to 5HT1A receptors on pyramidal glutamate neurons, an action that inhibits glutamate release. Additionally, serotonin binds to 5HT7 receptors on GABA interneurons in the prefrontal cortex. This stimulates GABA release, which in turn inhibits glutamate release.

Serotonin binding at 5HT7 receptors can also inhibit its own release. That is, when serotonergic neurons in the raphe nucleus are stimulated, they release serotonin throughout the brain, including not only in the prefrontal cortex but also in the raphe itself. Serotonin can then bind to 5HT7 receptors on GABA interneurons in the raphe nucleus. This stimulates GABA release, which then turns off serotonin release.

Serotonin binding at 5HT7 receptors in the raphe inhibits serotonin release; therefore, an antagonist at this receptor would be expected to enhance serotonin release. Specifically, by blocking serotonin from binding to the 5HT7 receptor on GABA interneurons, a 5HT7 antagonist would prevent the release of GABA onto serotonin neurons, thus allowing the continued release of serotonin in the prefrontal cortex.

References
Sarkisyan G, Roberts AJ, Hedlund PB. The 5-HT7 receptor as a mediator and modulator of antidepressant-like behavior. *Behav Brain Res* 2010;209(1):99–108.

Stahl SM. The serotonin-7 receptor as a novel therapeutic target. *J Clin Psychiatry* 2010;71(11):1414–5.

Unipolar Depression and Antidepressants

QUESTION SEVENTEEN

A 32-year-old woman with major depressive disorder has been taking a selective serotonin reuptake inhibitor (SSRI) with good response for 9 months. She presents now with complaints that she feels numb, and that even when she's sad she can't cry. Her clinician is considering reducing the dose of her SSRI in an effort to alleviate this problem. Is this a reasonable option?

A. Yes, data suggest that SSRI-induced indifference is dose-dependent and can be alleviated by reducing the dose

B. No, although data suggest that SSRI-induced indifference is dose-dependent, patients who develop this side effect generally require a switch to a different medication

C. No, SSRI-induced indifference is not dose-dependent and thus cannot be alleviated by reducing the dose

Answer to Question Seventeen

The correct answer is A.

Choice	Peer answers
Yes, data suggest that SSRI-induced indifference is dose-dependent and can be alleviated by reducing the dose	70%
No, although data suggest that SSRI-induced indifference is dose-dependent, patients who develop this side effect generally require a switch to a different medication	22%
No, SSRI-induced indifference is not dose-dependent and thus cannot be alleviated by reducing the dose	7%

A – Correct. Apathy and emotional blunting can be symptoms of depression, but they are also side effects associated with selective serotonin reuptake inhibitors (SSRIs). These symptoms – termed "SSRI-induced indifference" – are under-recognized but can be very distressing for patients. They are theoretically due to an increase in serotonin levels and a consequent reduction of dopamine release. The first recommended strategy for addressing SSRI-induced indifference is to lower the SSRI dose, if feasible. Additional options include adding an augmenting agent, or switching to an antidepressant in another class.

B and C – Incorrect.

References

Sansone RA, **Sansone LA**. SSRI-induced indifference. *Psychiatry (Edgemont)* 2010;7(1):14–8.

Stahl SM. *Case studies: Stahl's essential psychopharmacology*. New York, NY: Cambridge University Press; 2011.

Stahl SM. *Stahl's essential psychopharmacology*, fourth edition. New York, NY: Cambridge University Press; 2013. (Chapter 7)

Stahl SM. *Stahl's essential psychopharmacology, the prescriber's guide*, sixth edition. New York, NY: Cambridge University Press; 2017.

QUESTION EIGHTEEN

The hypothesis that the therapeutic effects of antidepressants are due to downstream changes in neuroplasticity is consistent with the fact that clinical improvement with antidepressants is typically delayed by several weeks. The downstream effects of monoamine antidepressants include:

A. Decreased AMPA receptor expression, decreased NMDA receptor expression, decreased glutamate

B. Increased AMPA receptor expression, decreased NMDA receptor expression, decreased glutamate

C. Decreased AMPA receptor expression, increased NMDA receptor expression, decreased glutamate

D. Increased AMPA receptor expression, decreased NMDA receptor expression, increased glutamate

Answer to Question Eighteen

The correct answer is B.

Choice	Peer answers
Decreased AMPA receptor expression, decreased NMDA receptor expression, decreased glutamate	10%
Increased AMPA receptor expression, decreased NMDA receptor expression, decreased glutamate	44%
Decreased AMPA receptor expression, increased NMDA receptor expression, decreased glutamate	21%
Increased AMPA receptor expression, decreased NMDA receptor expression, increased glutamate	25%

A – Incorrect. AMPA receptor expression is increased.

B – Correct. There is increasing evidence that the underlying mechanism of antidepressant treatment may not be alterations in the levels of monoamines themselves, but rather changes in the downstream molecular events and neuroplasticity triggered by those monoamines. Monoaminergic antidepressants likely exert their therapeutic effects by influencing downstream signaling, such as increased α-amino-3-hydroxy-5-methyl-4-isoxazolepropionic acid, or AMPA receptor expression, decreased N-methyl-D-aspartate, or NMDA receptor expression, and decreased glutamate, suggesting agents with direct activity at these downstream targets may lead to faster treatment response. Antidepressant treatments may modify the AMPA:NMDA receptor ratio, resulting in downregulated NMDA receptors, and increased AMPA receptors.

C – Incorrect. NMDA receptor expression is decreased.

D – Incorrect. Glutamate is decreased.

References

Abdallah CG, Adams TG, Kelmendi B, Esterlis I, Sanacora G, Krystal JH. Ketamine's mechanism of action: a path to rapid-acting antidepressants. *Depress Anxiety* 2016;33(8):689–97.

Barbon A, Caracciolo L, Orlandi C, et al. Chronic antidepressant treatments induce a time-dependent up-regulation of AMPA receptor subunit protein levels. *Neurochem Int* 2011;59(6):896–905.

Bunney BG, Bunney WE. Rapid-acting antidepressant strategies: mechanisms of action. *Int J Neuropsychopharmacol* 2012;15(5):695–713.

Racagni G, **Popoli M**. Cellular and molecular mechanisms in the long-term action of antidepressants. *Dialogues Clin Neurosci* 2008;10(4):385–400.

Stahl SM. *Stahl's essential psychopharmacology*, fourth edition. New York, NY: Cambridge University Press; 2013.

QUESTION NINTEEN

A 24-year-old woman with depression has just had genetic testing, including testing of the genes for catechol-O-methyltransferase (COMT) and methylenetetrahydrofolate reductase (MTHFR). Her symptoms are theoretically consistent with severe dopamine deficiency with apathy, anhedonia, psychomotor retardation, and cognitive slowing. Based on current literature, what genetic testing results might be most likely?

A. COMT Val/Val and MTHFR (T/T) or (C/T)

B. COMT Val/Val and MTHFR (C/C)

C. COMT Met/Met and MTHFR (T/T) or (C/T)

D. COMT Met/Met and MTHFR (C/C)

Unipolar Depression and Antidepressants

Answer to Question Nineteen

The correct answer is A.

Choice	Peer answers
COMT Val/Val and MTHFR (T/T) or (C/T)	40%
COMT Val/Val and MTHFR (C/C)	21%
COMT Met/Met and MTHFR (T/T) or (C/T)	30%
COMT Met/Met and MTHFR (C/C)	9%

The COMT gene contains a highly functional and common variation (position 472, guanine to adenine substitution) that causes a valine to methionine change in peptide sequence of COMT enzyme at codon 108/158 (val108/158 met). This results in COMT enzyme activity that is significantly reduced:

Allele	Met/Met	Met/Val	Val/Val
Activity	low	intermediate	high

The prefrontal cortex has few dopamine transporters; thus, dopamine inactivation in the prefrontal cortex is more dependent upon COMT metabolism. Therefore, when COMT activity is high (as with COMT158 Val), there is decreased dopamine in the prefrontal cortex, which in turn can be associated with cognitive deficits.

MTHFR is the predominant enzyme that converts inactive folic acid to an active form of folate. The 677T allele is associated with decreased MTHFR activity, leading to increased homocysteine and decreased methylation capacity. This can increase expression of COMT and lead to reduced dopamine.

Decreased methylation of COMT, caused by decreased function with the MTHFR 677T variant, hypothetically results in decreased dopamine signaling and may ultimately lead to cognitive impairments. This effect could hypothetically be exacerbated in patients who carry both the MTHFR 677T allele and the high–activity COMT 158 Val/Val genotype, with increased cognitive impairment. This effect has been demonstrated in schizophrenic patients but not in healthy controls.

A – Correct. Carrying both the COMT 158 Val/Val and the MTHFR 677 (T/T) or (C/T) genotypes theoretically would result in increased degradation of dopamine in the prefrontal cortex, leading to decreased dopamine signaling and associated cognitive dysfunction, apathy, and psychomotor retardation ("prefrontal dopamine" hypothesis).

B – Incorrect. COMT158Val/Val would theoretically result in decreased dopamine; however, MTHFR (C/C) would not.

C – Incorrect. COMT158 Met/Met would theoretically result in *decreased* degradation of dopamine, and thus *increased* dopamine signaling.

D – Incorrect.

References

Baune B, Hohoff C, Berger K et al. Association of the COMT val158met variant with antidepressant treatment response in major depression. *Neuropsychopharmacology* 2008;33:924–32.

Kato M, Serretti A. Review and meta-analysis of antidepressant pharmacogenetic findings in major depressive disorder. *Mol Psychiatry* 2010;15:473–500.

Kirchheiner J, Nickchen K, Bauer M et al. Pharmacogenetics of antidepressants and antipsychotics: the contribution of allelic variations to the phenotype of drug response. *Mol Psychiatry* 2004;9:442–73.

Kocabas NA, Faghel C, Barreto M et al. The impact of catechol-O-methyltransferase SNPs and haplotypes on treatment response phenotypes in major depressive disorder: a case–control association study. *Int Clin Psychopharmacol* 2010;25(4):218–27.

Nutt D, Demyttenaere K, Janka Z et al. The other face of depression, reduced positive affect: the role of catecholamines in causation and cure. *J Psychopharmacol* 2006;21(5):461–71.

Unipolar Depression and Antidepressants

QUESTION TWENTY

The labels for antidepressants (selective serotonine reupate inhibitors (SSRIs) in particular) include several warning statements about possible adverse effects of use during pregnancy. Which of the following has the most evidence suggesting an increased risk with antidepressant use during pregnancy?

A. First-trimester cardiac malformations

B. Persistent pulmonary hypertension of the newborn (PPHN)

C. Postnatal adaptation syndrome (PNAS)

D. Long-term neurodevelopmental abnormalities

Answer to Question Twenty

The correct answer is C.

Choice	Peer answers
First-trimester cardiac malformations	18%
Persistent pulmonary hypertension of the newborn (PPHN)	22%
Postnatal adaptation syndrome (PNAS)	56%
Long-term neurodevelopmental abnormalities	4%

A – Incorrect. The evidence for increased risk of first-trimester major malformations with antidepressants has been limited and inconsistent. Paroxetine, which carries a warning and a Pregnancy Risk Category of D, has shown increased risk of major and cardiac malformations in several studies, although this has not been seen in large database assessments. Limited data with bupropion has also shown possible increased risk of congenital heart defects. The results of these studies suggest that any increase in the absolute risk of cardiac malformations with antidepressant use is small. Consistent with this, a recent large, population-based cohort study did not identify a substantial increase in risk of cardiac malformations (relative risk vs. women with untreated depression was 1.06).

B – Incorrect. Persistent pulmonary hypertension of the newborn (PPHN) is a rare condition with a baseline risk of 1.9 per 1000 live births. Nonetheless, PPHN is fatal in approximately 20% of cases and is thus a serious concern. A recent meta-analysis has shown that although antidepressant (SSRI) use in late pregnancy does increase the risk for PPHN, the absolute risk remains small (4.75–5.40 per 1000 live births). The number needed to harm (NNH) in the meta-analysis was 286–351 – in other words, an additional 286–351 women would need to be treated with an SSRI in late pregnancy in order for one additional case of PPHN to occur.

C – Correct. Postnatal adaption syndrome (PNAS) in infants is characterized by irritability, abnormal crying, tremor, lethargy, hypoactivity, decreased feeding, tachypnea, and respiratory distress. Although there is some conflicting evidence, overall, data suggest that PNAS can occur in 20–30% of infants exposed to serotonergic antidepressants. PNAS has most often been reported with paroxetine, fluoxetine, or venlafaxine, but could theoretically occur with any antidepressant.

D – Incorrect. The data regarding the risk of long-term neurodevelopmental abnormalities with prenatal antidepressant are very limited. No studies have found detrimental effects on cognitive development. Two studies have found possible effects on motor developments. Overall, the existing studies are reassuring, but have limitations: most do not follow children through school age, control for maternal IQ, or measure maternal treatment adherence.

References

Byatt N, Deligiannidis KM, Freeman MP. Antidepressant use in pregnancy: a critical review focused on risks and controversies. *Acta Psychiatr Scand* 2013;127:94–114.

Gentile S, Galbally M. Prenatal exposure to antidepressant medications and neurodevelopmental outcomes: a systematic review. *J Affective Disord* 2011;128:1–9.

Grigoriadis S, Vonderporten EH, Mamisashvili L et al. Prenatal exposure to antidepressants and persistent pulmonary hypertension of the newborn: systematic review and meta-analysis. *BMJ* 2014;348:f6932.

Huybrechts KF, Palmsten K, Avorn J et al. Antidepressant use in pregnancy and the risk of cardiac defects. *N Engl J Med* 2014;370(25): 2397–407.

Unipolar Depression and Antidepressants

QUESTION TWENTY ONE

Sasha is a 58-year-old patient with a history of depression who has been prescribed agomelatine. At present, she is relatively free of depressive symptoms, likely due in part to binding of agomelatine to what receptors in the suprachiasmatic nucleus?

A. Melatonin receptors

B. Serotonin 2C receptors

C. Melatonin and serotonin 2C receptors

Answer to Question Twenty One

The correct answer is C.

Choice	Peer answers
Melatonin receptors	14%
Serotonin 2C receptors	14%
Melatonin and serotonin 2C receptors	71%

A and B – Partially correct.

C – Correct. Agomelatine is both a melatonin M1 and M2 receptor agonist and a serotonin 5HT2C receptor antagonist. This unique receptor profile gives agomelatine the ability to address impairments in neurotransmission as well as circadian rhythm dysfunction. First, agomelatine can modulate circadian rhythms through its agonist actions at melatonin receptors. Melatonin is normally released from the pineal gland in response to environmental cues. It then acts on the suprachiasmatic nucleus, the location of the master clock, to reset circadian rhythms. Thus, as an agonist at melatonin receptors, agomelatine likewise regulates the molecular clock and can resynchronize circadian rhythms that are disturbed in depression.

Second, agomelatine affects neurotransmission by blocking 5HT2C receptors. Normally, serotonin excites GABA interneurons by stimulating 5HT2C receptors, which increases the release of the inhibitory neurotransmitter GABA. GABA can then bind to GABA-A receptors on noradrenergic and dopaminergic neurons. Because GABA is inhibitory, it will prevent these neurons from releasing norepinephrine and dopamine in the prefrontal cortex. As a 5HT2C receptor antagonist, agomelatine blocks serotonin from binding to GABA interneurons. This leads to disinhibition of monoaminergic neurons and increased norepinephrine and dopamine in the prefrontal cortex, which could potentially improve mood and cognition.

References
DeBodinat C, Guardiola-Lemaitre B, Mocaer E et al. Agomelatine, the first melatonergic antidepressant: discovery, characterization, and development. *Nature Reviews Drug Discov* 2010;9:628–42.

CHAPTER PEER COMPARISON

For the Unipolar Depression section, the correct answer was selected 62% of the time.

4 BIPOLAR DISORDER AND MOOD STABILIZERS

QUESTION ONE

A 34-year-old man has recently been diagnosed with bipolar disorder, 6 years after his symptoms began. He has had no mood-stabilizing treatment in that time. According to the kindling model and allostatic load hypothesis, what progressive pattern of illness would you expect this patient to have exhibited over the course of the last 6 years?

A. Longer interval between episodes, worsened emotionality, minimal change in cognitive impairment

B. Shorter interval between episodes, worsened emotionality, minimal change in cognitive impairment

C. Longer interval between episodes, worsened emotionality, worsened cognitive impairment

D. Shorter interval between episodes, worsened emotionality, worsened cognitive impairment

Answer to Question One

The correct answer is D.

Choice	Peer answers
Longer interval between episodes, worsened emotionality, minimal change in cognitive impairment	2%
Shorter interval between episodes, worsened emotionality, minimal change in cognitive impairment	18%
Longer interval between episodes, worsened emotionality, worsened cognitive impairment	4%
Shorter interval between episodes, worsened emotionality, worsened cognitive impairment	77%

A, B, and C – Incorrect.

D – Correct. Throughout the course of illness, patients with bipolar disorder will experience manic or hypomanic episodes, depressive episodes, and inter-episode periods during which they are generally well but may have subsyndromal symptoms. The pattern of episodes can differ for each patient; however, in general the clinical course of bipolar disorder is progressive. That is, as the number of episodes a person has had increases, the **interval between episodes gets shorter** and **emotionality may worsen**. In addition, **cognitive impairment seems to worsen** with the length of illness. Increasing episode number is also associated with reduced likelihood of treatment response.

Models for how these changes may come to be posit that recurrent mood episodes are associated with repeated physiological insults that add up and kindle, like a spark bursting into fire. This could compromise endogenous compensatory mechanisms, leading to cell apoptosis that in turn causes rewiring of the brain circuits involved in mood regulation and cognition. This can render one more vulnerable to the effects of stressors, increasing risk of future episodes and thus perpetuating the vicious spiral.

References

Berk M, Kapczinski F, Andreazza AC et al. Pathways underlying neuroprogression in bipolar disorder: focus on inflammation, oxidative stress, and neurotrophic factors. *Neurosci Biobehav Rev* 2011;35(3): 804–17.

Kapczinksi F, Vieta E, Andreazza AC et al. Allostatic load in bipolar disorder: implications for pathophysiology and treatment. *Neurosci Biobehav Rev* 2008;32:675–92.

Post RM. Kindling and sensitization as models for affective episode recurrence, cyclicity, and tolerance phenomena. *Neurosci Biobehav Rev* 2007;31:858–73.

Bipolar Disorder and Mood Stabilizers

QUESTION TWO

A 28-year-old woman with bipolar disorder recently began taking a mood stabilizer and has experienced improvement in her symptoms. Which of the following are mechanisms by which different mood stabilizers may prevent mitochondrial dysfunction in bipolar disorder?

A. Increasing levels of anti-apoptotic proteins

B. Decreasing levels of pro-apoptotic proteins

C. Increasing levels of key antioxidants

D. A and B

E. A, B, and C

Answer to Question Two

The correct answer is E.

Choice	Peer answers
Increasing levels of anti-apoptotic proteins	6%
Decreasing levels of pro-apoptotic proteins	5%
Increasing levels of key antioxidants	3%
A and B	21%
A, B, and C	65%

Mitochondria are intracellular organelles that regulate energy through cell respiration. They also play critical roles in regulating cell apoptosis. Mitochondrial dysfunction can therefore contribute to inappropriate cell damage and death.

There are multiple ways in which mitochondrial dysfunction can lead to apoptosis. Mitochondria contain both pro- and anti-apoptotic proteins that must remain in a delicate balance to control the integrity of the mitochondrial membrane. If that balance is shifted, this can cause morphological changes to the mitochondrial membrane, allowing the release of cytochrome C and other substances that induce apoptosis.

One factor that may shift the balance of pro- and anti-apoptotic proteins is an excess of free radicals, which themselves are produced by mitochondria during cell respiration. Normally, antioxidant defenses in the brain can stabilize the free radicals, thus creating oxidative balance. If antioxidants are depleted, then free radicals may accumulate and activate pro-apoptotic proteins, thus initiating the mitochondrial pathway of apoptosis.

A, B, C, and D – Incorrect.

E – Correct. Both lithium and valproate have been shown to **increase levels of the anti-apoptotic protein** Bcl-2, thus maintaining the balance of pro- and anti-apoptotic proteins, restoring the integrity of the mitochondrial membrane, and preventing release of cytochrome C. Some atypical antipsychotics may **reduce elevated levels of the pro-apoptotic protein Bax**. Lithium and valproate have both been shown **to increase levels of the antioxidant glutathione**, which may help reduce the presence of free radicals and thus prevent activation of the mitochondrial pathway of apoptosis.

References

Bachman RF, **Wang Y**, **Yuan P** et al. Common effects of lithium and valproate on mitochondrial functions: protection against methamphetamine-induced mitochondrial damage. *Int J Neuropsychopharmacol* 2009;12:805–22.

Berk M, **Kapczinski F**, **Andreazza AC** et al. Pathways underlying neuroprogression in bipolar disorder: focus on inflammation, oxidative stress, and neurotrophic factors. *Neurosci Biobehav Rev* 2011;35(3): 804–17.

Hunsberger J, **Austin DR**, **Henter ID**, **Chen G**. The neurotrophic and neuroprotective effects of psychotropic agents. *Dialogues Clin Neurosci* 2009;11(3):333–48.

Bipolar Disorder and Mood Stabilizers

QUESTION THREE

A 32-year-old woman with bipolar I disorder has just found out that she is 6 weeks pregnant. Her mania has been stable on a combination of lithium, valproate, and quetiapine, but she is unsure about the safety of maintaining her medications during her pregnancy. Which of the following is true regarding the use of these medications for bipolar disorder during pregnancy?

A. Lithium has known teratogenic effects and is not a preferred treatment

B. Lithium and valproate have known teratogenic effects and are not preferred treatments

C. Lithium, valproate, and quetiapine have known teratogenic effects and are not preferred treatments

Answer to Question Three

The correct answer is B.

Choice	Peer answers
Lithium has known teratogenic effects and is not a preferred treatment	3%
Lithium and valproate have known teratogenic effects and are not preferred treatments	86%
Lithium, valproate, and quetiapine have known teratogenic effects and are not preferred treatments	12%

A – Incorrect. Lithium has known teratogenic effects, but so does valproate.

B – Correct. Both lithium and valproate have known teratogenic effects. Lithium has evidence of increased risk of major birth defects and cardiac anomalies, especially Ebstein's anomaly, although a recent review suggested that the risk of cardiac anomalies may be overemphasized. Valproate is associated with increased risk of neural tube defects (e.g., spina bifida) and other congenital anomalies.

C – Incorrect. Quetiapine does not have known teratogenic effects. If quetiapine or another atypical antipsychotic is used during pregnancy, weight gain and the risk for gestational diabetes should be more carefully monitored, with glucose tolerance testing (as opposed to glucose challenge testing) at 14–16 weeks and again at 28 weeks. After delivery, infants should be monitored for neonatal withdrawal, toxicity, extrapyramidal side effects (EPS), and sedation.

References

Galbally M, Snellen M, Power J. Antipsychotic drugs in pregnancy: a review of their maternal and fetal effects. *Therapeutic Adv Drug Safety* 2014;5(2):100–9.

Gentile S. Antipsychotic therapy during early and late pregnancy. A systematic review. *Schizophr Bull* 2010;36(3):518–44.

Stahl SM. *Stahl's essential psychopharmacology: the prescriber's guide*, sixth edition. New York, NY: Cambridge University Press; 2017.

Yacobi S, Ornoy A. Is lithium a real teratogen? What can we conclude from the prospective versus retrospective studies? A review. *Isr J Psychiatry Relat Sci* 2008;45(2):95–106.

Bipolar Disorder and Mood Stabilizers

QUESTION FOUR

A 28-year-old woman presents with a depressive episode. She has previously been hospitalized and treated for a manic episode but is not currently taking any medication. The agents with the strongest evidence of efficacy in bipolar depression are:

A. Lamotrigine, lithium, quetiapine

B. Quetiapine, olanzapine–fluoxetine, lurasidone

C. Olanzapine–fluoxetine, lurasidone, lamotrigine

D. Lurasidone, lamotrigine, lithium

Bipolar Disorder and Mood Stabilizers

Answer to Question Four

The correct answer is B.

Choice	Peer answers
Lamotrigine, lithium, quetiapine	19%
Quetiapine, olanzapine–fluoxetine, lurasidone	51%
Olanzapine–fluoxetine, lurasidone, lamotrigine	16%
Lurasidone, lamotrigine, lithium	14%

A – Incorrect. Controlled data assessing the efficacy of lithium in bipolar depression are too limited to draw conclusions; empiric evidence suggests that this agent may not be as effective in the depressed phase as in the manic phase or for maintenance treatment. Lithium does have evidence for reducing suicidality, however. Lamotrigine has been tested in more trials than lithium, but a recent meta-analysis failed to support its efficacy.

B – Correct. Quetiapine, olanzapine–fluoxetine, and lurasidone have all demonstrated consistent efficacy in bipolar depression and are approved for this stage of the disorder.

Drug	Daily dose
Lurasidone	20–120 mg
Olanzapine–fluoxetine	6–12/25–50 mg
Quetiapine	300 mg

C – Incorrect. Consistent evidence of efficacy does not exist for lamotrigine.

D – Incorrect. Consistent evidence of efficacy does not exist for lamotrigine or lithium.

References

Nivoli AMA, Colom F, Murru A et al. New treatment guidelines for acute bipolar depression. A systematic review. *J Affect Disord* 2010;129:14–26.

Selle V, Schalkwijk S, Vazquez GH, Baldessarini RJ. Treatments for acute bipolar depression: meta-analyses of placebo-controlled, monotherapy trials of anticonvulsants, lithium and antipsychotics. *Pharmacopsychiatry* 2014;47(2):43–52.

QUESTION FIVE

A 24-year-old female patient, who recently moved from Germany, presents to your office during a manic episode that initiated following abrupt discontinuation of her medication as she ran out of her prescription. She informs you that she had been diagnosed with rapid-cycling bipolar disorder, and wants to be prescribed the same medication she used to take in Germany but does not remember the generic name of the medication. She gives you the following information: she was on 1250 mg/day; she gained weight when she started it, which she did not like, but she liked the sedating effects of the drug, which helped calm her down and sleep at night. Her German doctor had told her she could experience the following side effects: hair loss, hepatotoxicity, and seizure upon abrupt withdrawal. Also she knows that she should consider switching medications when she intends to become pregnant, as the medication can lead to birth defects. Which medication was she most probably taking?

A. Lamotrigine

B. Gabapentin

C. Aripiprazole

D. Valproate

Answer to Question Five

The correct answer is D.

Choice	Peer answers
Lamotrigine	1%
Gabapentin	1%
Aripiprazole	1%
Valproate	97%

A – Incorrect. The dose range of **lamotrigine** is 100–200 mg/day, and lamotrigine does not generally induce sedation or weight gain, thus this is not the correct answer. Patients with epilepsy could seize upon abrupt discontinuation of lamotrigine, but this medication has no known teratogenic side effects and does not induce hepatotoxicity or hair loss. Lamotrigine seems to be more effective in treating depressive episodes than manic episodes in bipolar disorder.

B – Incorrect. The dose range of **gabapentin** is 900–1800 mg/day, and this medication does induce sedation, and upon rapid discontinuation it can lead to relapses in bipolar patients. However, hepatotoxicity is unusual with gabapentin, as is hair loss. Gabapentin is not known to be efficacious for bipolar disorder.

C – Incorrect. The dose range of **aripiprazole** is 15–30 mg/day. Additionally, aripiprazole does not normally induce weight gain or sedation, and has no known teratogenic effects.

D – Correct. **Valproate** is one of the first-line treatments for rapid-cycling bipolar disorder, and can induce all the side effects mentioned by the patient. The dose range is 1200–1500 mg/day for mania, and rapid discontinuation increases the risk of relapse.

References

Stahl SM. *Stahl's essential psychopharmacology*, fourth edition. New York, NY: Cambridge University Press; 2013. (Chapter 8)

Stahl SM. *Essential psychopharmacology, the prescriber's guide*, sixth edition. New York, NY: Cambridge University Press; 2017.

QUESTION SIX

A 17-year-old girl presents with symptoms of depression. She has always been a good student and a caring and responsible sister to her two younger siblings. Recently, she has suddenly become somewhat withdrawn and reports feeling sad much of the time. Her MADRS score is 35, indicating severe depression. This patient also endorses feelings of hostility and aggression and has recently started getting into physical altercations with her peers. There is no information regarding family history, as the patient is adopted. Although not definitive, this particular symptom profile may be more suggestive of:

A. Unipolar depression

B. Bipolar depression

Answer to Question Six

The correct answer is B.

Choice	Peer answers
Unipolar depression	16%
Bipolar depression	84%

A – Incorrect. Data to date suggest that, although in no way definitive, there may be certain symptoms and course-related factors that help differentiate between unipolar and bipolar depression. This patient's presentation, which includes rapid and early onset of severe depression, hostility, aggression, and impulsivity, raises the suspicion that this may be part of a bipolar illness rather than a unipolar illness.

B – Correct. The patient's presentation includes multiple factors that may be more likely to occur with bipolar disorder rather than with unipolar depression. This is not definitive, but does suggest caution when making treatment decisions. Although also not definitive, family history and input from someone close to the patient are generally more valuable than specific symptoms.

Suspect bipolar depression if:
Positive family history of bipolar disorder
*Early onset of first depressive episode (<25 years)
Greater # of lifetime affective episodes
Postpartum depressive episodes
*Rapid onset of depressive episodes
*Greater severity of depressive episodes
Worse response to antidepressants
Antidepressant-induced hypomania
Psychotic features
Atypical depressive symptoms (e.g., leaden paralysis)
*Impulsivity
*Aggression
*Hostility

(cont.)

Suspect bipolar depression if:
Comorbid substance use disorder

References

Angst J, Azorin JM, Bowden CL et al. Prevalence and characteristics of undiagnosed bipolar disorders in patients with a major depressive episode: the BRIDGE study. *Arch Gen Psychiatry* 2011;68(8):791–9.

Dervic K, Garcia–Amador M, Sudol K et al. Bipolar I and II versus unipolar depression: clinical differences and impulsivity/aggression traits. *Eur Psychiatry* 2015;30(1):106–13.

Bipolar Disorder and Mood Stabilizers

QUESTION SEVEN

The "bipolar storm" refers to the concept that unstable, unregulated and excessive neurotransmission occurs at synapses in specific brain regions, and both voltage-sensitive sodium channels and voltage-sensitive calcium channels are involved in this excessive stimulation of glutamate release. Which drugs would theoretically reduce glutamate release by blocking voltage-sensitive sodium channels?

A. Valproate and lamotrigine

B. Pregabalin and gabapentin

C. Levetiracetam and amantadine

STAHL'S SELF-ASSESSMENT EXAMINATION IN PSYCHIATRY

Answer to Question Seven

The correct answer is A.

Choice	Peer answers
Valproate and lamotrigine	86%
Pregabalin and gabapentin	11%
Levetiracetam and amantadine	3%

A – Correct. **Valproate** is a nonspecific voltage-sensitive sodium channel modulator and **lamotrigine** also blocks voltage-sensitive sodium channels, hypothesized to lead to reduction in glutamate release.

B – Incorrect. **Pregabalin** and **gabapentin** are alpha 2 delta ligands at voltage-sensitive calcium channels, which also lead to reduction in glutamate release.

C – Incorrect. **Levetiracetam** is a modulator of the synaptic vesicle protein SV2A, and **amantadine** is an antagonist of the NDMA receptor. While this combination of drugs would lead to reduced glutamate release, it would not do so via the mechanisms of action asked.

References

Sitges M, Chiu LM, Guarneros A, Nekrassov V. Effects of carbamazepine, phenytoin, lamotrigine, oxcarbazepine, topiramate, and vinpocetine on NA+ channel-mediated release of [3H]glutamate in hippocampal nerve endings. *Neuropharmacology* 2007;52(2):598–605.

Stahl SM. *Stahl's essential psychopharmacology*, fourth edition. New York, NY: Cambridge University Press; 2013. (Chapter 8)

QUESTION EIGHT

A 24-year-old man has been taking lithium for 3 years to treat his bipolar disorder. What are two primary candidates for the direct mechanisms of lithium?

A. Inhibition of glycogen synthase kinase 3β (GSK-3β) and inositol monophosphatase (IMPase)

B. Activation of GSK-3β and IMPase

C. Inhibition of GSK-3β and activation of IMPase

D. Activation of GSK-3β and inhibition of IMPase

Answer to Question Eight

The correct answer is A.

Choice	Peer answers
Inhibition of glycogen synthase kinase 3β (GSK-3β) and inositol monophosphatase (IMPase)	58%
Activation of GSK-3β and IMPase	5%
Inhibition of GSK-3β and activation of IMPase	24%
Activation of GSK-3β and inhibition of IMPase	14%

A – Correct. Lithium has been a first-line treatment for bipolar disorder for decades, yet its mechanism of action is still not certain. There is, however, substantial evidence that lithium exerts neuroprotective effects that are likely downstream from its primary mode of action. Two primary candidates for the direct mechanisms of lithium are the inhibition of glycogen synthase kinase 3β (GSK-3β) and the inhibition of inositol monophosphatase (IMPase). GSK-3β is involved in the regulation of inflammation and is, in general, pro-apoptotic. Specifically, it inhibits transcription factors that would otherwise induce production of cytoprotective proteins such as brain-derived neurotrophic factor (BDNF); thus, its inhibition may be neuroprotective. IMPase indirectly leads to an increase in protein kinase C, which is overactive in mania. Thus, inhibition of IMPase by lithium could potentially reduce manic symptoms.

B – Incorrect. Lithium is thought to inhibit GSK-3β and IMPase, not activate them.

C – Incorrect. Lithium is thought to inhibit IMPase, not activate it.

D – Incorrect. Lithium is thought to inhibit GSK-3β, not activate it.

References

Chu CT, Chuang DM. Molecular actions and therapeutic potential of lithium in preclinical and clinical studies of CNS disorders. *Pharmacol Ther* 2010;128:281–304.

Pasquali L, Busceti CL, Fulceri F, Paparelli A, Fornai F. Intracellular pathways underlying the effects of lithium. *Behav Pharmacol* 2010;21: 473–92.

Quiroz JA, Machado-Vieira R, Zarate Jr CA, Manji HK. Novel insights into lithium's mechanism of action: neurotrophic and neuroprotective effects. *Neuropsychobiology* 2010;62:50–60.

QUESTION NINE

A 24-year-old man with bipolar disorder is being initiated on lithium, with monitoring of his levels until a therapeutic serum concentration is achieved. Once the patient is stabilized, how often should his serum lithium levels be monitored (excluding one-off situations such as dose or illness change)?

A. Every 2–3 months

B. Every 6–12 months

C. Every 1–2 years

D. Routine monitoring is not necessary

Answer to Question Nine

The correct answer is B.

Choice	Peer answers
Every 2–3 months	19%
Every 6–12 months	79%
Every 1–2 years	1%
Routine monitoring is not necessary	1%

A – Incorrect. Initially, lithium levels should be monitored every 1–2 weeks until the desired serum concentration is achieved, and then every 2–3 months for the first 6 months. However, this frequency of monitoring is not required once the patient is stabilized.

B – Correct. Once a patient is stabilized, lithium levels need only be monitored every 6–12 months.

C – Incorrect (every 1–2 years).

D – Incorrect (routine monitoring is not necessary).

References

Grandjean EM, Aubry JM. Lithium: updated human knowledge using an evidence-based approach. Part II: Clinical pharmacology and therapeutic monitoring. *CNS Drugs* 2009;23(4):331–49.

McKnight RF, Adida M, Budge K et al. Lithium toxicity profile: a systematic review and meta-analysis. *Lancet* 2012;379:721–8.

QUESTION TEN

A 49-year-old clerk with bipolar disorder has been maintained on 900 mg/day of lithium. She was doing well for a long time and had even been able to lose the weight she had initially gained with lithium. She broke up with her boyfriend 5 months ago and has been feeling depressed ever since. You augment her with 300 mg/day of quetiapine, but after several weeks she complains of weight gain and wants to change medications. Blockade of which two receptors was most likely responsible for this weight gain induced by quetiapine?

A. Serotonin 2A and muscarinic 3

B. Dopamine 2 and alpha 1 adrenergic

C. Muscarinic 1 and serotonin 6

D. Serotonin 2C and histamine 1

Answer to Question Ten

The correct answer is D.

Choice	Peer answers
Serotonin 2A and muscarinic 3	11%
Dopamine 2 and alpha 1 adrenergic	8%
Muscarinic 1 and serotonin 6	1%
Serotonin 2C and histamine 1	80%

A – Incorrect. Blockade of **serotonin 2A** receptors is considered a beneficial property of antipsychotics leading to fewer extrapyramidal symptoms. Blockade of **muscarinic M3** receptors has been linked to inducing cardiometabolic risk, but has not been linked to weight gain per se.

B – Incorrect. **Dopamine 2** blockade is the main property of antipsychotics and, if continuous, this blockade can lead to motor side effects, but not to weight gain. **Alpha 1 blockade** can result in decreased blood pressure, dizziness, and drowsiness, but does not lead to weight gain.

C – Incorrect. Blockade of **muscarinic M1 receptors** can lead to constipation, blurred vision, dry mouth, and drowsiness, but not weight gain. The function of the **serotonin 6** receptors has not been identified yet.

D – Correct. Blockade of **serotonin 2C** receptors and **histamine 1** receptors has been linked to weight gain.

References

Kroeze WK, **Hufeisen SJ**, **Popadak BA** et al. H1-histamine receptor affinity predicts short-term weight gain for typical and atypical antipsychotic drugs. *Neuropsychopharmacology* 2003;28(3):519–26.

Stahl SM. *Stahl's essential psychopharmacology*, fourth edition. New York, NY: Cambridge University Press; 2013. (Chapters 5, 8)

Stahl SM, **Mignon L**. *Stahl's illustrated antipsychotics*, second edition. New York, NY: Cambridge University Press; 2009.

QUESTION ELEVEN

Maria is a 31-year-old patient with bipolar II disorder. During major depressive episodes, this patient often experiences several symptoms of hypomania, including flight of ideas, increased risk-taking behavior, and increased talkativeness. According to data from the Stanley Foundation Bipolar Network, how many patients with bipolar disorder exhibit subsyndromal hypomanic symptoms during a major depressive episode?

A. 5%

B. 25%

C. 45%

D. 65%

E. 85%

Answer to Question Eleven

The correct answer is D.

Choice	Peer answers
5%	3%
25%	36%
45%	25%
65%	36%
85%	1%

A, B, C, and E – Incorrect.

D – Correct. According to data published by the Stanley Foundation Bipolar Network, as many as 65% of patients with bipolar disorder exhibit symptoms of subsyndromal hypomania during depressive episodes.

References

Miller S, Suppes T, Mintz J et al. Mixed depression in bipolar disorder: prevalence rate and clinical correlates during naturalistic follow-up in the Stanley Bipolar Network. *Am J Psychiatry* 2016;173(10):1015–23.

QUESTION TWELVE

A 43-year-old obese patient with bipolar II disorder has agreed to a trial of an atypical antipsychotic. Considering this patient's current weight and the wish to avoid any treatment-induced weight gain, which of the following treatments would be the **least** optimal treatment for this patient?

A. Lurasidone

B. Olanzapine

C. Aripiprazole

Answer to Question Twelve

The correct answer is B.

Choice	Peer answers
Lurasidone	8%
Olanzapine	84%
Aripiprazole	8%

A and C – Incorrect. Among atypical antipsychotics, lurasidone and aripiprazole have relatively benign profiles in adults in terms of cardiometabolic effects; both lurasidone and aripiprazole have little to no risk of either weight gain or dyslipidemia.

B – Correct. Although olanzapine is approved for the treatment of bipolar depression, mania, and maintenance, among the atypical antipsychotics olanzapine carries with it one of the highest risks for cardiometabolic side effects, including weight gain.

References
Stahl SM. *Stahl's essential psychopharmacology*, fourth edition. New York, NY: Cambridge University Press; 2013. (Chapter 5)

Stahl SM. *Essential psychopharmacology, the prescriber's guide*, sixth edition. New York, NY: Cambridge University Press; 2017.

QUESTION THIRTEEN

Thomas, a 28-year-old patient with major depressive disorder with mixed features, complains of significant irritability and agitation that are affecting his family and work. Which psychotropic treatment(s) can be considered as ALTERNATIVE maintenance treatments to antidepressants?

A. An atypical antipsychotic such as quetiapine

B. A mood stabilizer such as lamotrigine

C. A benzodiazepine such as lorazepam

D. A and B only

E. B and C only

Answer to Question Thirteen

The correct answer is D.

Choice	Peer answers
An atypical antipsychotic such as quetiapine	10%
A mood stabilizer such as lamotrigine	4%
A benzodiazepine such as lorazepam	0%
A and B only	85%
B and C only	2%

A – Partially correct. Atypical antipsychotics with mood–stabilizing properties (such as quetiapine) are recommended as first–line treatments in patients with major depressive disorder with mixed features.

B – Partially correct. Mood stabilizers (such as lamotrigine) are recommended as first– or second–line treatments in patients with major depressive disorder with mixed features.

C and E – Incorrect. Although benzodiazepines (such as lorazepam) may be useful for reducing acute mania, there are no data supporting the use of benzodiazepines in the maintenance treatment of major depressive disorder with mixed features. Additionally, the extended use of benzodiazepines is not recommended due to high risk for dependence, tolerance, and withdrawal.

D – Correct. Both atypical antipsychotics with mood–stabilizing properties and mood stabilizers have shown some efficacy in the treatment of major depressive episodes with mixed features and are therefore recommended as first– or second–line treatments.

References

McIntyre RS, Lee Y, Mansur RB. A pragmatic approach to the diagnosis and treatment of mixed features in adults with mood disorders. *CNS Spectr* 2016;21:28–32.

Stahl SM. *Essential psychopharmacology, the prescriber's guide*, sixth edition. New York, NY: Cambridge University Press; 2017.

Stahl SM, Morrissette DA, Faedda G et al. Guidelines for the recognition and treatment of mixed depression. *CNS Spectr* 2017;22(2): 203–19.

QUESTION FOURTEEN

Ten-year-old Rebecca experienced seizures as a toddler. Her mother took her to a psychiatrist at age 8, because she had violent outbursts of anger, was attacking her older brother, and was severely irritable. That behavior had been going on for the last 6 months. After screening her for ADHD, and other conduct disorders, Dr. Jones had diagnosed her with bipolar I disorder and put her on 800 mg/day of carbamazepine. Over the last few years she has only had a couple of manic episodes but has recently started having frequent debilitating migraines. She has gained weight as well, and now weighs 30 kg (height of 100 cm, BMI = 30) and her mother does not want her to start a medication that could lead to more weight gain. Which medication, and at which dose, could be added to her current treatment?

A. 150 mg/day of topiramate (= 5 mg/kg/day)

B. 400 mg/day of topiramate (= 13 mg/kg/day)

C. 900 mg/day of lithium

D. 1800 mg/day of lithium

E. 10 mg/day of olanzapine

F. 30 mg/day of olanzapine

Answer to Question Fourteen

The correct answer is A.

Choice	Peer answers
150 mg/day of topiramate (= 5 mg/kg/day)	90%
400 mg/day of topiramate (= 13 mg/kg/day)	5%
900 mg/day of lithium	3%
1800 mg/day of lithium	0%
10 mg/day of olanzapine	1%
30 mg/day of olanzapine	0%

A – Correct. Besides being used off-label as an adjunct in bipolar disorder, **topiramate** is FDA approved as an antimigraine medication. It has no weight gain potential, and might even lead to weight loss. Children should be given a lower dose than adults, and the normal dose range for children is 5–9 mg/kg/day.

B – Incorrect. This **dose** of topiramate is too high for children.

C and D – Incorrect. **Lithium** can be used for vascular headaches, but is not recommended in children, and children tend to have more frequent and severe side effects on lithium. Additionally, lithium can cause weight gain, which is a side effect that the mother wishes to avoid.

E and F – Incorrect. The antipsychotic **olanzapine**, while a good adjunct to carbamazepine for breakthrough manic episodes, is highly likely to induce weight gain, and would therefore not be the medication of choice.

References

Stahl SM. *Stahl's essential psychopharmacology*, fourth edition. New York, NY: Cambridge University Press; 2013. (Chapter 8)

Stahl SM. *Stahl's essential psychopharmacology, the prescriber's guide*, sixth edition. New York, NY: Cambridge University Press; 2017.

QUESTION FIFTEEN

A 23-year-old patient with major depressive disorder presents with several symptoms that may indicate the presence of mixed features. Which of the following symptoms was NOT excluded from the DSM-5 mixed features specifier diagnostic criteria?

A. Agitation

B. Irritability

C. Increased goal-directed activity

D. Distractibility

Answer to Question Fifteen

The correct answer is C.

Choice	Peer answers
Agitation	8%
Irritability	22%
Increased goal-directed activity	62%
Distractibility	8%

A, B, and D – Incorrect. Although irritability, distractibility, and psychomotor agitation are among the most common symptoms of DMX, they are excluded from DSM-5 mixed features criteria due to the overlap of these symptoms with other disorders (e.g., anxiety disorders) and between mania and depression

C – Correct. Although increased goal-directed activity is not one of the most common symptoms exhibited by patients experiencing a major depressive episode with mixed features, it is included in the DSM-5 mixed features specifier diagnostic criteria.

References

Koukopoulos A, Sani G. DSM-5 criteria for depression with mixed features: a farewell to mixed depression. *Acta Psychiatr Scand* 2014;129:4–16.

Mahli GS, Laampe L, Coulston CM et al. Mixed state discrimination: a DSM problem that won't go away? *J Affective Disord* 2014;158:8–10.

Takeshima M, Oka T. DSM-5-defined 'mixed features' and Benazzi's mixed depression: which is practically useful to discriminate bipolar disorder from unipolar depression in patients with depression? *Psychiatry Clin Neurosci* 2015;69(2):109–16.

QUESTION SIXTEEN

A patient with bipolar depression has been treated for 6 months with lamotrigine plus an atypical antipsychotic with partial response. The decision is made to stop the atypical antipsychotic; however, during downtitration, the patient develops withdrawal dyskinesias. No treatment for the dyskinesias is initiated, and after 2 weeks, they still remain. Which of the following is true?

A. If the withdrawal dyskinesias still remain after 2 weeks, they are likely to be permanent

B. The patient's withdrawal dyskinesias may take several weeks to months to resolve

Answer to Question Sixteen

The correct answer is B.

Choice	Peer answers
If the withdrawal dyskinesias still remain after 2 weeks, they are likely to be permanent	10%
The patient's withdrawal dyskinesias may take several weeks to months to resolve	90%

A – Incorrect. Withdrawal dyskinesias are often reversible with time and usually resolve within a few weeks; however, they can take several months to resolve, depending on their seriousness. Thus, although the patient's withdrawal dyskinesias still remain after 2 weeks, this does not indicate that they are likely to be permanent.

B – Correct. It may take several weeks to months for the patient's withdrawal dyskinesias to resolve.

References

Aia PG, Reveulta GJ, Cloud LJ, Factor SA. Tardive dyskinesia. *Curr Treatment Options Neurol* 2011;13(3):231–41.

Moseley CN, Simpson-Khanna HA, Catalano G, Catalano MC. Covert dyskinesia associated with aripiprazole: a case report and review of the literature. *Clin Neuropharmacol* 2013;36(4):128–30.

Umbrich P, Soares KV. Benzodiazepines for neuroleptic-induced tardive dyskinesia. *Cochrane Database Syst Rev* 2003;(2):CD000205.

QUESTION SEVENTEEN

A patient with bipolar disorder has been taking valproate with only partial control of depressive symptoms, and his clinician elects to add lamotrigine. Compared to lamotrigine monotherapy, what adjustment should be made to the lamotrigine titration schedule in the presence of valproate?

A. Slower titration schedule, same target dose

B. Same titration schedule, half the target dose

C. Slower titration schedule, half the target dose

D. Same titration schedule, same dose

Answer to Question Seventeen

The correct answer is C.

Choice	Peer answers
Slower titration schedule, same target dose	6%
Same titration schedule, half the target dose	18%
Slower titration schedule, half the target dose	72%
Same titration schedule, same dose	3%

A, B, and D – Incorrect.

C – Correct. Valproate increases the plasma levels of lamotrigine, so when adding lamotrigine to valproate the target dose is lower and titration is slower (in comparison to initiating lamotrigine monotherapy):

- For the first 2 weeks: 25 mg every other day
- Week 3: increase to 25 mg/day
- Week 5: increase to 50 mg/day
- Week 6: increase to 100 mg/day

References

Stahl SM. *Essential psychopharmacology, the prescriber's guide*, sixth edition. New York, NY: Cambridge University Press; 2017.

QUESTION EIGHTEEN

A 28-year-old obese woman presents with a depressive episode. She has previously been hospitalized and treated for a manic episode but is not currently taking any medication. The agent with the lowest risk of cardiometabolic side effects is:

A. Lithium

B. Lurasidone

C. Valproate

Answer to Question Eighteen

The correct answer is B.

Choice	Peer answers
Lithium	11%
Lurasidone	82%
Valproate	7%

A and C – Incorrect. Both lithium and valproate are associated with a relatively high risk of significant weight gain.

B – Correct. Among atypical antipsychotics, lurasidone has a relatively benign profile in terms of cardiometabolic effects. In fact, many patients who are switched to lurasidone from a previous psychotropic agent associated with weight gain experience a reversal in cardiometabolic effects.

References

Stahl SM. *Stahl's essential psychopharmacology, the prescriber's guide*, sixth edition. New York, NY: Cambridge University Press; 2017.

QUESTION NINTEEN

Michael is a 42-year-old patient with bipolar I disorder who frequently exhibits impulsive symptoms of mania including risk-taking and pressured speech during his manic episodes. Compared to a healthy brain, neuroimaging of this patient's brain during a no-go task (designed to test response inhibition) would likely show:

A. Increased activity in the orbitofrontal cortex

B. Decreased activity in the orbitofrontal cortex

C. Increased activity in the dorsolateral prefrontal cortex

Answer to Question Ninteen

The correct answer is B.

Choice	Peer answers
Increased activity in the orbitofrontal cortex	25%
Decreased activity in the orbitofrontal cortex	54%
Increased activity in the dorsolateral prefrontal cortex	21%

A – Incorrect. Compared to healthy controls, neuroimaging studies indicate that the orbitofrontal cortex is hypoactive while performing a no-go task in patients with mania.

B – Correct. Neuroimaging of the orbitofrontal cortex of manic patients during a no-go task (a task that required the patient to suppress a response) shows that they fail to appropriately activate this brain region. This neuroimaging anomaly suggests that patients with bipolar disorder have problems with impulsivity associated with mania and with the orbitofrontal cortex.

C – Incorrect. Neuroimaging studies indicate that resting activity in the dorsolateral prefrontal cortex of depressed patients is decreased compared to healthy controls. However, there are no data indicating an elevation in activity in the dorsolateral prefrontal cortex during a no-go task in manic patients. In fact, research indicates that patients with bipolar disorder show reduced activity in the dorsolateral prefrontal cortex in response to fearful faces.

References

Elliot R, Ogilvie A, Rubinsztein JS, Calderon G et al. Abnormal ventral frontal response during performance of an affective go/no go task in patients with mania. *Biol Psychiatry* 2004;155(12):1163–70.

Price JL, Drevets WC. Neurocircuitry of mood disorders. *Neuropsychopharmacology* 2010;35(1):192–216.

Stahl SM. *Stahl's essential psychopharmacology*, fourth edition. New York, NY: Cambridge University Press; 2013. (Chapter 6)

QUESTION TWENTY

Sarah is a 20–year–old patient who presents with symptoms of depression (including sadness, feelings of worthlessness, and suicidal ideation) occurring every day for the past month. Clinical interview with Sarah reveals that she has a maternal aunt with bipolar disorder I. Further assessment reveals that this patient also feels distracted and as though her thoughts are racing. Upon speaking with the patient's mother, it is discovered that Sarah has been, at times, more talkative than usual and irritable with her friends and family. Which class of medication would NOT be recommended as monotherapy for this patient?

A. An antidepressant

B. A mood stabilizer

C. An antipsychotic

Answer to Question Twenty

The correct answer is A.

Choice	Peer answers
An antidepressant	98%
A mood stabilizer	1%
An antipsychotic	1%

A – Correct. Expert consensus and published guidelines recommend that antidepressant monotherapy **NOT** be used (and is contraindicated) in patients with depression who exhibit mixed features and a positive family history of bipolar disorder.

B – Incorrect. Expert consensus and published guidelines recommend that patients who exhibit mixed features during a major depressive episode and positive family history of bipolar disorder be treated with a mood stabilizer as a first- or second-line treatment strategy.

C – Incorrect. Expert consensus and published guidelines recommend that patients who exhibit mixed features during a major depressive episode and positive family history of bipolar disorder be treated with an atypical antipsychotic that has evidence of mood stabilizing properties (e.g., lurasidone, quetiapine) as a first- or second-line treatment strategy.

References
Stahl SM, Morrissette DA, Faedda G et al. Guidelines for the recognition and management of mixed depression. *CNS Spectrums* 2017;22(2):203–19.

QUESTION TWENTY ONE

Stacey is a 25-year-old patient with bipolar depression who tends to endorse some manic symptoms during depressive episodes. Of the following symptoms, which is the most common subsyndromal mania symptom in patients during a major depressive episode with mixed features?

A. Decreased need for sleep

B. Inflated self-esteem

C. Psychomotor agitation

D. Elevated mood

E. High-risk behavior

Answer to Question Twenty One

The correct answer is C.

Choice	Peer answers
Decreased need for sleep	22%
Inflated self-esteem	1%
Psychomotor agitation	68%
Elevated mood	1%
High-risk behavior	8%

A, B, D, and E – Incorrect. Decreased need for sleep, inflated self-esteem, elevated mood, and high-risk behavior are among the manic symptoms most rarely seen in patients with mixed features during a major depressive episode.

C – Correct. During a major depressive episode with mixed features (concomitant subthreshold levels of mania or hypomania), the most common manic/hypomanic symptom exhibited is psychomotor agitation.

References

Koukopoulos A, Sani G. DSM-5 criteria for depression with mixed features: a farewell to mixed depression. *Acta Psychiatr Scand* 2014;129:4–16.

Mahli GS, Laampe L, Coulston CM et al. Mixed state discrimination: a DSM problem that won't go away? *J Affective Disord* 2014;158:8–10.

Takeshima M, Oka T. DSM-5-defined 'mixed features' and Benazzi's mixed depression: which is practically useful to discriminate bipolar disorder from unipolar depression in patients with depression? *Psychiatry Clin Neurosci* 2015;69(2):109–16.

CHAPTER PEER COMPARISON

For the Bipolar Disorders section, the correct answer was selected 71% of the time.

5 ANXIETY DISORDERS AND ANXIOLYTICS

QUESTION ONE

A 35-year-old female presents to your office and begins to divulge her frequent worries: ever since she was young she was worried someone close to her would die in a freak accident. As she grew older, this worry was exacerbated by the fear that she would pass away without telling her friends and family how important they are to her. Additionally, once she had children, she became so worried for their safety that she rarely lets them leave the house. Furthermore, she has constant worries about how things will work out for her in the future, and recently experienced a panic attack. How might you currently diagnose this patient?

A. Posttraumatic stress disorder

B. Panic disorder

C. Social anxiety disorder

D. Generalized anxiety disorder

Answer to Question One

The correct answer is D.

Choice	Peer answers
Posttraumatic stress disorder	0%
Panic disorder	4%
Social anxiety disorder	0%
Generalized anxiety disorder	96%

A – Incorrect. Posttraumatic stress disorder generally originates after a traumatic event; it does not appear that this patient has ever actually experienced a traumatic death experience. She just appears to have excessive worry.

B – Incorrect. Panic disorder is characterized by the presence of spontaneous panic attacks, which this patient does not report having.

C – Incorrect. Worry in social anxiety disorder is tied to embarrassment, whereas this patient's worry is related to a fear of dying.

D – Correct. This patient is displaying core symptoms of generalized anxiety disorder via generalized anxiety and worry. Although she did have a panic attack, a single panic attack is insufficient for a diagnosis of either panic disorder or social anxiety disorder.

References

Stahl SM. *Stahl's essential psychopharmacology*, fourth edition. New York, NY: Cambridge University Press; 2013.

Stahl SM, Grady MM. *Stahl's illustrated anxiety, stress, and PTSD*. New York, NY: Cambridge University Press; 2010.

QUESTION TWO

Which part of the central fear response system at the core of the fear response is associated with increased startle response?

A. Lateral hypothalamus

B. Midbrain central gray

C. Parabrachial nucleus

D. N. reticularis pontis caudalis

E. Trigeminal/facial motor nerve

F. Lateral tegmental nucleus

Answer to Question Two

The correct answer is D.

Choice	Peer answers
Lateral hypothalamus	29%
Midbrain central gray	15%
Parabrachial nucleus	12%
N. reticularis pontis caudalis	29%
Trigeminal/facial motor nerve	1%
Lateral tegmental nucleus	14%

A – Incorrect. The lateral hypothalamus is associated with sympathetic activation in the central fear response system.

B – Incorrect. The midbrain central gray is associated with freezing and fear of dying in the central fear response system.

C – Incorrect. The parabrachial nucleus is associated with dyspnea/hyperventilation in the central fear response system

D – Correct. The N. reticularis pontis caudalis is associated with increased startle response in the central fear response system.

E – Incorrect. The trigeminal/facial motor nerve is associated with facial expression of fear in the central fear response system.

F – Incorrect. The lateral tegmental nucleus is associated with increased vigilance in the central fear response system.

References

Kandel ER, Schwartz JH, Jessell TM, Siegelbaum SA, Hudspeth AJ. *Principles of neural science*, fifth edition. Columbus, OH: McGraw-Hill Education; 2012.

Shin LM, Liberzon I. The neurocircuitry of fear, stress, and anxiety disorders. *Neuropsychopharmacology* 2010;35(1): 169–91.

Steimer T. The biology of fear- and anxiety-related behaviors. *Dialogues Clin Neurosci* 2002;4(3):231–49.

QUESTION THREE

A 46-year-old female patient has been experiencing several anxiety-based symptoms for many years, and was previously diagnosed with generalized anxiety disorder. She describes difficulty concentrating in addition to difficulty falling asleep. Her family has recently told her that she seems to be displaying heightened anger responses toward them over minor details. Oftentimes she will cry for extended periods of time and become irritable and distant. Based on the above patient's revelations, if she were to continue to experience these stressful reactions to stimuli (i.e., excessive crying, fatigue, problems concentrating, tension, irritability), what could potentially occur?

A. Increased hippocampal volume

B. Reduced brain-derived neurotrophic factor (BDNF) production

C. Reduced reactivity to stress

D. Decreased hippocampal volume

E. B and D

F. A and C

Answer to Question Three

The correct answer is E.

Choice	Peer answers
Increased hippocampal volume	2%
Reduced brain-derived neurotrophic factor (BDNF) production	5%
Reduced reactivity to stress	1%
Decreased hippocampal volume	4%
B and D	84%
A and C	3%

A and C – Incorrect. Hippocampal volume in chronic stress is actually theorized to decrease, not increase. Reduced reactivity to stress may occur in patients who experience mild stressors while growing up, which may result in an improved adaptability when dealing with adult stressors. However, severe or persistent stress, such as this adult is experiencing, does not lead to reduced reactivity to stress.

B and D – Correct. Reduced BDNF production can occur in patients who experience chronic stress, leading to a decreased ability to create and maintain neurons and neuronal connections. Decreased hippocampal volume, perhaps related to decreased expression of BNDF, has been reported in some chronic stress conditions such as major depression and certain anxiety disorders. A major treatment strategy for stress-related disorders is the use of selective serotonin reuptake inhibitors (SSRIs), which can increase BDNF levels because serotonin initiates signal transduction cascades that lead to BDNF release.

E – Correct; as both B and D are correct answers.

F – Incorrect; as both A and C are incorrect answers.

References

Bremner JD. Stress and brain atrophy. *CNS Neurol Disord Drug Targets* 2006;5(5):503–12.

Stahl SM, **Grady MM**. *Stahl's illustrated anxiety, stress, and PTSD*. New York, NY: Cambridge University Press; 2010.

QUESTION FOUR

A 51-year-old male veteran with chronic postraumatic stress disorder (PTSD) has agreed to begin pharmacotherapy for his debilitating symptoms of arousal and anxiety associated with his experiences in Iraq 2 years ago. Which of the following would be appropriate as first-line treatment?

A. Paroxetine

B. Paroxetine or lorazepam

C. Paroxetine, lorazepam, or D-cycloserine

D. Paroxetine, lorazepam, D-cycloserine, or quetiapine

Answer to Question Four

The correct answer is A.

Choice	Peer answers
Paroxetine	90%
Paroxetine or lorazepam	5%
Paroxetine, lorazepam, or D-cycloserine	2%
Paroxetine, lorazepam, D-cycloserine, or quetiapine	3%

A – Correct. Paroxetine, a selective serotonin norepinephrine reuptake inhibitor, is approved for use in posttraumatic stress disorder (PTSD).

B – Incorrect. Lorazepam is a benzodiazepine. Benzodiazepines do not have evidence of efficacy in PTSD and are not generally recommended for first-line use in PTSD.

C – Incorrect. D-Cycloserine, an NMDA agonist, has been theorized to be useful in facilitating fear extinction, and may be useful in conjunction with exposure therapy. However, it is not a first-line choice.

D – Incorrect. Quetiapine, an atypical antipsychotic, is not approved as first-line treatment for PTSD, but may be useful in selected cases as a third-line treatment, specifically for sleep and possible reduction of nightmares.

References

Sauve W, **Stahl SM**. Psychopharmacological treatment of PTSD. In: *Treating PTSD in military personnel: a clinical handbook*. New York, NY: Guilford Press; 2011.

Stahl SM. *Case studies: Stahl's essential psychopharmacology*. New York, NY: Cambridge University Press; 2011.

Stahl SM, **Grady MM**. *Stahl's illustrated anxiety, stress, and PTSD*. New York, NY: Cambridge University Press; 2010.

QUESTION FIVE

A 34-year-old woman with posttraumatic stress disorder has been treated with exposure therapy, with partial success. Her clinician is considering an adjunct medication. The agent D-cycloserine could be efficacious for reducing symptoms in anxiety disorders because it has been shown to:

A. Modulate glutamate neurotransmission during fear conditioning

B. Modulate glutamate neurotransmission during fear extinction

Answer to Question Five

The correct answer is B.

Choice	Peer answers
Modulate glutamate neurotransmission during fear conditioning	27%
Modulate glutamate neurotransmission during fear extinction	73%

A – Incorrect. When an individual encounters a stressful or fearful experience, the sensory input is relayed to the amygdala, where it is integrated with input from the ventromedial prefrontal cortex (VMPFC) and hippocampus, so that a fear response can be either generated or suppressed. The amygdala may "remember" stimuli associated with that experience by increasing the efficiency of glutamate neurotransmission, so that on future exposure to stimuli, a fear response is more efficiently triggered. If this is not countered by input from the VMPFC to suppress the fear response, fear conditioning proceeds. Because D-cycloserine, as an N-methyl-D-aspartate (NMDA) co-agonist, may strengthen the efficiency of glutamate neurotransmission, it would theoretically *increase* rather than decrease the likelihood of fear conditioning.

B – Correct. Fear conditioning is not readily reversed, but it can be inhibited through new learning. This new learning is termed fear extinction and is the progressive reduction of the response to a feared stimulus that is repeatedly presented without adverse consequences. Thus the VMPFC and hippocampus learn a new context for the feared stimulus and send input to the amygdala to suppress the fear response. The "memory" of the conditioned fear is still present, however. Strengthening of synapses involved in fear extinction could help enhance the development of fear extinction learning in the amygdala and reduce symptoms of anxiety disorders. Administration of the D-cycloserine while an individual is receiving exposure therapy could increase the efficiency of glutamate neurotransmission at synapses involved in fear extinction.

References

Stahl SM. *Stahl's essential psychopharmacology: the prescriber's guide*, sixth edition. New York, NY: Cambridge University Press; 2017.

QUESTION SIX

A 26-year-old patient with panic disorder is willing to begin pharmacotherapy for treatment of his phobias and panic attacks. Clonazepam is suggested; what would be your recommended dose?

A. 0.25 mg/day to begin, uptitrating to 1 mg/day after 3 days

B. 4 mg/day, uptitrating to 6 mg/day after 1 week

C. 2 mg/day, uptitrating every 3 days until 20 mg/day is reached

D. 1.5 mg/day, uptitrating 0.5 mg/day every other day

Answer to Question Six

The correct answer is A.

Choice	Peer answers
0.25 mg/day to begin, uptitrating to 1 mg/day after 3 days	88%
4 mg/day, uptitrating to 6 mg/day after 1 week	2%
2 mg/day, uptitrating every 3 days until 20 mg/day is reached	2%
1.5 mg/day, uptitrating 0.5 mg/day every other day	8%

A – Correct. For panic disorder, the general recommended dose is 0.25 mg/day divided into 2 doses, raised 1 mg after 3 days dosed twice daily or once at bedtime.

B – Incorrect. Maximum dose is generally 4 mg/day for panic disorder, not the starting dose.

C – Incorrect. 2 mg/day is not the general recommended starting dose for panic disorder. Additionally, 20 mg/day is the maximum dose for seizures, not panic disorder.

D – Incorrect. 1.5 mg/day is generally the starting dose recommended for seizures, not panic disorder.

References

Stahl SM. *Stahl's essential psychopharmacology: the prescriber's guide*, sixth edition. New York, NY: Cambridge University Press; 2017.

QUESTION SEVEN

A 4-year-old girl has just been removed from her home by social services due to suspicions of abuse and neglect. Severe early life stress can cause changes in functioning of the hypothalamic pituitary adrenal (HPA) axis, which in turn can increase risk for the development of future stress-related disorders. Research suggests that modulation at what level may be necessary in order to prevent the changes in HPA functioning that occur with early stress?

A. Corticotropin-releasing hormone (CRH) gene expression/ CRH activity

B. Adrenocorticotropic hormone (ACTH) gene expression/ ACTH activity

C. Cortisol gene expression/cortisol activity

Answer to Question Seven

The correct answer is A.

Choice	Peer answers
Corticotropin-releasing hormone (CRH) gene expression/CRH activity	58%
Adrenocorticotropic hormone (ACTH) gene expression/ACTH activity	20%
Cortisol gene expression/cortisol activity	22%

A – Correct. Changes in HPA axis functioning that can occur with severe early life stress may begin with the *Crh* gene. That is, changes in *Crh* gene expression precede the other changes that are seen with early mild or severe stress. Thus, in cases of mild stress, it seems that reduced expression of CRH promotes less peptide release in response to stress, and therefore less glucocorticoid release, which ultimately causes upregulation of glucocorticoid receptors. In addition, studies with non-handled rats show that blocking CRH from binding to its type 1 receptor can lead to the same changes and corresponding enhancements in cognitive function. Similarly, blocking CRH1 receptors soon after exposure to early-life chronic stress can normalize hippocampal function in adulthood.

The results of these studies suggest that some of the mechanisms behind the risk for stress-related disorders may be set in motion at a very young age. Accordingly, treatment may need to be administered not after symptoms develop, but rather immediately after – or during – exposure to early life stress, in order to prevent the changes in gene expression that may confer greater risk later in life. This may explain why CRH1 antagonists in major depressive disorder in adults – long after possible exposure to early life stressors – have been mostly ineffective.

B, C, and D – Incorrect.

References
Korosi A, **Baram TZ**. Plasticity of the stress response early in life: mechanisms and significance. *Dev Psychobiol* 2010;52:661–70.

McClelland S, **Korosi A**, **Cope J**, **Ivy A**, **Baram TZ**. Emerging roles of epigenetic mechanisms in the enduring effects of early-life stress and experience on learning and memory. *Neurobiol Learning Mem* 2011;96(1):79–88.

QUESTION EIGHT

A 31-year-old female assault victim is brought to the emergency room after tracking down passersby for help. She appears rightly traumatized from the incident. Which of the following pharmacotherapy options has been theorized as a potential pre-emptive treatment to the development of posttraumatic stress disorder (PTSD)?

A. *N*-methyl-D-aspartate (NMDA) agonist such as D-cycloserine

B. Alpha 2 delta ligand such as pregabalin

C. Beta adrenergic blocker such as propranolol

D. Benzodiazepine such as diazepam

Answer to Question Eight

The correct answer is C.

Choice	Peer answers
N-methyl-D-aspartate (NMDA) agonist such as D-cycloserine	23%
Alpha 2 delta ligand such as pregabalin	4%
Beta adrenergic blocker such as propranolol	68%
Benzodiazepine such as diazepam	5%

A – Incorrect. An NMDA agonist is useful in facilitating fear extinction, but would most likely not be helpful in this case, as the trauma has just occurred.

B – Incorrect. Alpha 2 delta ligands may be used off-label in the USA to treat anxiety, but are often utilized once the disorder has been diagnosed, rather than dealing with an immediate trauma. Preemptive treatment has produced some potentially promising results, if administered within the appropriate window of time from trauma.

C – Correct. Beta adrenergic blockers have been shown to block formation of fear conditioning immediately following trauma. Thus, in this case, propranolol may be theoretically useful (off-label) to aid in decreasing risk of developing an anxiety disorder like PTSD due to her incident.

D – Incorrect. Benzodiazepines are commonly used to treat established anxiety disorders, rather than to pre-empt the development of an anxiety disorder.

References

Orr SP, Milad MR, Metzger LJ, Lasko NB, Gilbertson MW, Pitman RK. Effects of beta blockade, PTSD diagnosis, and explicit threat on the extinction and retention of an aversively conditioned response. *Biol Psychol* 2006;732:262–71.

Sauve W, Stahl SM. Psychopharmacological treatment of PTSD. In: *Treating PTSD in military personnel: a clinical handbook*. New York, NY: Guilford Press; 2011.

Stahl SM. *Case studies: Stahl's essential psychopharmacology*. New York, NY: Cambridge University Press; 2011.

Stahl SM, Grady MM. *Stahl's illustrated anxiety, stress, and PTSD*. New York, NY: Cambridge University Press; 2010.

QUESTION NINE

Sarah is a 24-year old patient with generalized anxiety disorder. She is taking a benzodiazepine and has been complaining of sleepiness associated with taking the medication. Which GABA-A alpha subunit has been most associated with sedation properties of benzodiazepines?

A. GABA-A receptors containing alpha-1 subunits

B. GABA-A receptors containing alpha-2 subunits

C. GABA-A receptors containing alpha-3 subunits

D. GABA-A receptors containing alpha-4 subunits

Answer to Question Nine

The correct answer is A.

Choice	Peer answers
GABA-A receptors containing alpha-1 subunits	42%
GABA-A receptors containing alpha-2 subunits	39%
GABA-A receptors containing alpha-3 subunits	13%
GABA-A receptors containing alpha-4 subunits	5%

Currently available benzodiazepines are nonselective for GABA-A receptors with different alpha subunits. Benzodiazepines bind to GABA-A alpha subunits: alpha 1, alpha 2, alpha 3, and alpha 5. Each of these subunits is associated with different effects, and thus benzodiazepines not only cause sedation but are also anxiolytic, cause muscle relaxation, and have alcohol potentiating actions.

A – Correct. Benzodiazepine-sensitive GABA-A receptors with alpha-1 subunits may be most important for regulating sleep and are the presumed targets of numerous sedative–hypnotic agents.

B and C – Incorrect. Benzodiazepine-sensitive GABA-A receptors with alpha-2 subunits and alpha-3 subunits may be most important for regulating anxiety and are the presumed targets of anxiolytic benzodiazepine.

D – Incorrect. GABA-A receptors containing alpha-4 subunits are benzodiazepines-insensitive, are located extrasynaptically, and regulate tonic inhibition.

References

Nuss P. Anxiety disorders and GABA neurotransmission: a disturbance of modulation. *Neuropsychiatr Dis Treat* 2015;11:165–75.

Stahl SM. Selective actions on sleep or anxiety by exploiting GABA-A/benzodiazepine receptor subtypes. *J Clin Psychiatry* 2002;63(3):179–80.

Stahl SM. *Stahl's essential psychopharmacology*, fourth edition. New York, NY: Cambridge University Press; 2013.

QUESTION TEN

A man who was severely bitten by a dog as a child is beginning cognitive restructuring therapy to treat his posttraumatic stress disorder (PTSD). He identifies walking down the sidewalk past a person with their dog on a leash as a highly distressing situation, rating his fear during such an encounter as 80/100. He states that he strongly believes any dog is likely to escape its leash and attack him. The next step in cognitive restructuring would be for him to:

A. Put himself in a situation in which he encounters a dog on a leash

B. Identify evidence for and against the thought that the dog would escape and attack him

C. Practice techniques such as breathing exercises while thinking about encountering a dog on a leash

Answer to Question Ten

The correct answer is B.

Choice	Peer answers
Put himself in a situation in which he encounters a dog on a leash	3%
Identify evidence for and against the thought that the dog would escape and attack him	70%
Practice techniques such as breathing exercises while thinking about encountering a dog on a leash	28%

A – Incorrect. Putting himself in a situation in which he encounters his fear (i.e., a dog) would be part of exposure therapy, but is not part of cognitive restructuring.

B – Correct. Cognitive restructuring is a process by which patients learn to evaluate and modify inaccurate and unhelpful thoughts (e.g., "All dogs are vicious"). There are six main steps of cognitive restructuring: (1) identify a distressing event/thought; (2) identify and rate (0–100) emotions related to the event/thought; (3) identify automatic thoughts associated with the emotions, rate the degree to which one believes them, and select one to challenge; (4) identify evidence in support of and against the thought; (5) generate a response to the thought using the evidence for/against (even though <evidence for>, in fact <evidence against>) and rate the degree of belief in the response; and (6) rerate emotion related to the event/thought.

C – Incorrect. Breathing exercises are not part of cognitive restructuring.

References

Forneris CA, Gartlehner G, Brownley KA, et al. Interventions to prevent post-traumatic stress disorder: a systematic review. *Am J Prev Med* 2013;44(6):635–50.

Kliem S, Kroger C. Prevention of chronic PTSD with early cognitive behavioral therapy. A metaanalysis using mixed-effects modeling. *Behav Res Ther* 2013;51(11):753–61.

Stahl SM, Grady MM. *Stahl's illustrated anxiety, stress, and PTSD*. New York, NY: Cambridge University Press; 2010.

Zayfert C, Becker CB. *Cognitive-behavioral therapy for PTSD: a case formulation approach*. New York, NY: The Guildford Press; 2007.

QUESTION ELEVEN

A 39-year-old veteran presents with comorbid posttraumatic stress disorder (PTSD) and substance abuse. Her care provider recommends addressing her PTSD and substance use disorder (SUD) simultaneously. Which of the following statements is true regarding managing co-occurring PTSD and SUD?

A. Individualized trauma-focused PTSD treatment, like Prolonged Exposure, alongside SUD intervention can reduce PTSD severity and drug/alcohol use

B. Non-trauma-focused PTSD therapies, like Seeking Safety, are more effective than treatment as usual for reducing PTSD symptoms in patients with PTSD and SUD

C. The presence of a SUD should prevent concurrent treatment and SUD must be stabilized prior to treating the PTSD

Answer to Question Eleven

The correct answer is A.

Choice	Peer answers
Individualized trauma-focused PTSD treatment, like Prolonged Exposure, alongside SUD intervention can reduce PTSD severity and drug/alcohol use	62%
Non-trauma-focused PTSD therapies, like Seeking Safety, are more effective than treatment as usual for reducing PTSD symptoms in patients with PTSD and SUD	23%
The presence of a SUD should prevent concurrent treatment and SUD must be stabilized prior to treating the PTSD	15%

A – Correct. Individual trauma-focused PTSD therapies that have a primary component of exposure and/or cognitive restructuring, like Prolonged Exposure, when delivered together with SUD interventions, were more likely than SUD treatment alone or treatment as usual to improve PTSD symptoms in individuals with co-occurring PTSD and SUD. Patients with PTSD and SUD can tolerate and benefit from evidence-based trauma-focused PTSD treatment such as Prolonged Exposure.

B – Incorrect. Non-trauma-focused PTSD therapies (e.g., Seeking Safety), when delivered together with a SUD therapy, do not improve PTSD symptoms in individuals with SUDs more than SUD treatment alone or treatment as usual. Non-trauma-focused therapies such as Seeking Safety for the treatment of PTSD in the context of co-occurring SUD is not recommended.

C – Incorrect. Recent research has shown that patients with PTSD and SUD (including nicotine use disorder) can both tolerate and benefit from concurrent treatment for both conditions, even in the most severe cases.

References

Management of Posttraumatic Stress Disorder Work Group. VA/DOD Clinical practice guideline: the management of posttraumatic stress disorder and acute stress reaction 2017. Washington DC; Department of Defense, 2017.

Roberts NP, Roberts PA, Jones N, Bisson JI. Psychological interventions for post-traumatic stress disorder and comorbid substance use disorder: a systematic review and meta-analysis. *Clin Psychol Rev* 2015;38:25–38.

Stahl SM, Grady MM. *Stahl's illustrated anxiety, stress, and PTSD*. New York, NY: Cambridge University Press; 2010.

Zandberg LJ, Rosenfield D, Mclean CP, Powers MB, Asnaani A, Foa EB. Concurrent treatment of posttraumatic stress disorder and alcohol dependence: predictors and moderators of outcome. *J Consult Clin Psychol* 2016;84(1):43–56.

Anxiety Disorders and Anxiolytics

QUESTION TWELVE

A 57-year-old man presents with depression and a history of obsessive compulsive symptoms that began in his twenties and are mostly religious in nature. He has not responded to numerous previous trials of serotonergic medications at typical depression doses. He fairly recently began cognitive-behavioral therapy and has responded well to it; however, he continues to experience significant symptoms of obsessive compulsive disorder (OCD), rating his symptoms a 7/10 in severity. His current medications include fluoxetine 80 mg/day and trazodone 50 mg/night. Which of the following is true regarding the appropriate dosing of selective serotonin reuptake inhibitors (SSRIs) in OCD?

A. Doses are typically lower than those in depression

B. Doses are typically the same as those in depression

C. Doses are typically higher than those in depression

Answer to Question Twelve

The correct answer is C.

Choice	Peer answers
Doses are typically lower than those in depression	6%
Doses are typically the same as those in depression	2%
Doses are typically higher than those in depression	92%

A – Incorrect (doses are typically lower than those in depression).

B – Incorrect (doses are typically the same as those in depression).

C – Correct. Higher doses of SSRIs than those used in depression are often needed in OCD, in many cases exceeding the recommended maximum dose:

Recommended daily doses for OCD	
Citalopram	40 mg*
Clomipramine	250 mg
Escitalopram	60 mg
Fluoxetine	120 mg
Fluvoxamine	450 mg
Paroxetine	100 mg
Sertraline	400 mg

*The previous recommended daily dose for citalopram in OCD was 120 mg/day; however, the label for citalopram now includes a warning that citalopram may cause QTc prolongation at doses above 40 mg/day.

References

Abudy A, Juven-Wetzler A, Zohar J. Pharmacological management of treatment-resistant obsessive-compulsive disorder. *CNS Drugs* 2011;25(7):585–96.

QUESTION THIRTEEN

Which of the following drugs can diminish anxiety but does NOT have sedative, hypnotic, anticonvulsant, or musculoskeletal relaxing activity?

A. Diazepam

B. Buspirone

C. Mirtazapine

D. Haloperidol

Answer to Question Thirteen

The correct answer is B.

Choice	Peer answers
Diazepam	0%
Buspirone	95%
Mirtazapine	2%
Haloperidol	3%

A – Incorrect. Diazepam is a benzodiazepine that is nonspecific and works by binding to multiple GABA-A receptors subtypes, including the alpha-1 subunit that is important for sedation

B – Correct. Buspirone is a serotonin 5-HT1A receptor partial agonist used to treat anxiety. Buspirone's partial agonist actions at presynaptic somatodendritic serotonin autoreceptors may theoretically enhance serotonergic activity and contribute to antidepressant actions. The partial agonist actions postsynaptically may theoretically diminish serotonergic activity and contribute to anxiolytic actions. It does not produce significant sedation, hypnotic, anticonvulsant, or musculoskeletal relaxing effects.

C – Incorrect. Mirtazapine blocks 5HT2A, 5HT2C, and 5HT3 serotonin receptors and blocks H1 histamine receptors. Histamine 1 receptor antagonism may explain sedative effects.

D – Incorrect. By blocking dopamine 2 receptors in the striatum, haloperidol can cause motor side effects. Also, by blocking alpha 1 adrenergic receptors, it can cause dizziness, sedation, and hypotension.

References

Manfredi RL, Kales A, Vgontzas AN, Bixler EO, Isaac MA, Falcone CM. Buspirone: sedative or stimulant effect? *Am J Psychiatry* 1991;148(9):1213–7.

Ramboz S, Oosting R, Amara DA, et al. Serotonin receptor 1A knockout: an animal model of anxiety-related disorder. *Proc Natl Acad Sci USA* 1998;95(24):14476–81.

Piszczek L, Piszczek A, Kuczmanska J, Audero E, Gross CT. Modulation of anxiety by cortical serotonin 1A receptors. *Front Behav Neurosci* 2015;9:48.

Stahl SM. *Stahl's essential psychopharmacology*, fourth edition. New York, NY: Cambridge University Press; 2013.

Stahl SM. *Stahl's essential psychopharmacology: the prescriber's guide*, sixth edition. New York, NY: Cambridge University Press; 2017.

QUESTION FOURTEEN

A 38-year-old man with a history of treatment-resistant PTSD has now experienced improvement on quetiapine 300 mg/day, duloxetine 90 mg/day, and zolpidem 10 mg at bedtime. However, he complains of ongoing nightmares and difficulty staying asleep. He was previously initiated on prazosin 3 mg at bedtime, but he experienced intolerable dizziness, and it was discontinued. Can this patient be rechallenged with prazosin? If so, at what dose?

A. Yes; dose should be initiated at 1 mg at bedtime

B. Yes; dose should be initiated at 3 mg at bedtime

C. No; prazosin is contraindicated with quetiapine

D. No; prazosin should not be reattempted in patients with previous intolerability

Answer to Question Fourteen

The correct answer is A.

Choice	Peer answers
Yes; dose should be initiated at 1 mg at bedtime	88%
Yes; dose should be initiated at 3 mg at bedtime	1%
No; prazosin is contraindicated with quetiapine	4%
No; prazosin should not be reattempted in patients with previous intolerability	7%

A – Correct. Prazosin, an alpha 1 antagonist, can be an effective treatment for nightmares in PTSD. The initial dose of prazosin should be 1 mg at bedtime and titrated up 1 mg every 2–3 days to decrease the risk of syncope.

B – Incorrect. There is risk of "first dose effect" syncope with sudden loss of consciousness (1%) with an initial dose of at least 2 mg; thus, 3 mg would be too high for an initiation dose.

C – Incorrect. Prazosin is not contraindicated with quetiapine. The only contraindications for prazosin are proven allergy to prazosin or to quinazolines (e.g., the cancer medications gefitinib and erlotinib or the prostatic hyperplasia medications alfuzosin and bunazosin).

D – Incorrect. There is no reason why a patient cannot be rechallenged with prazosin if they experienced previous intolerability (assuming they did not have an allergic reaction). Patients may require slower titration or lower dose if they have previously not tolerated prazosin.

References

Kung A, Espinel Z, Lalpid MI. Treatment of nightmares with prazosin: a systematic review. *Mayo Clin Proc* 2012;87(9):890–900.

Simon PY, Rousseau PF. Treatment of post-traumatic stress disorders with the alpha-1 adrenergic antagonist prazosin. *Can J Psychiatry* 2017;62(3):186–98.

Stahl SM. *Stahl's essential psychopharmacology: the prescriber's guide*, sixth edition. New York, NY: Cambridge University Press; 2017.

Anxiety Disorders and Anxiolytics

QUESTION FIFTEEN

A 28-year-old combat veteran with PTSD has not responded to multiple trials of oral medication. He suffers from nightmares, rarely maintains sleep longer than 2 hours, and has lost interest in his family life, which is particularly difficult for his wife given that she is pregnant with their first child. The role of glutamate in traumatic memory formation and extinction suggests that ketamine may be beneficial; however, the potential side-effect profile of ketamine could also be concerning for patients with PTSD. In a recent controlled proof-of-concept study in PTSD, ketamine:

A. Did not reduce PTSD symptoms and caused transient worsening of dissociative symptoms

B. Did not reduce PTSD symptoms and caused sustained worsening of dissociative symptoms

C. Reduced PTSD symptoms and caused transient worsening of dissociative symptoms

D. Reduced PTSD symptoms and caused sustained worsening of dissociative symptoms

Answer to Question Fifteen

The correct answer is C.

Choice	Peer answers
Did not reduce PTSD symptoms and caused transient worsening of dissociative symptoms	9%
Did not reduce PTSD symptoms and caused sustained worsening of dissociative symptoms	3%
Reduced PTSD symptoms and caused transient worsening of dissociative symptoms	82%
Reduced PTSD symptoms and caused sustained worsening of dissociative symptoms	6%

Like D-cycloserine, ketamine could theoretically strengthen the efficiency of glutamate neurotransmission at synapses involved in fear extinction and thus improve symptoms of PTSD. In a proof-of-concept, double-blind, randomized, crossover trial comparing ketamine to the active placebo control midazolam, researchers found that ketamine infusion was associated with significant reduction in PTSD symptom severity, assessed 24 hours after infusion. This remained significant after adjusting for depressive symptom severity. In the study, ketamine caused transient worsening of dissociative symptoms, but this was not sustained. The clinical relevance of this study will be subject both to successful replication and to identification of an alternate method of ketamine administration. Methods that are under investigation for depression include intranasal and intramuscular.

A – Incorrect. It is true that ketamine caused transient worsening of dissociative symptoms; however, it also reduced PTSD symptoms.

B – Incorrect. Ketamine caused transient but not sustained worsening of dissociative symptoms.

C – Correct. Ketamine reduced PTSD symptoms and caused transient worsening of dissociative symptoms.

D – Incorrect (reduced PTSD symptoms and caused sustained worsening of dissociative symptoms).

References

Feder A, **Parides MK**, **Murrough JW** et al. Efficacy of intravenous ketamine for treatment of chronic posttraumatic stress disorder: a randomized clinical trial. *JAMA Psychiatry* 2014;71(6):681–8.

Womble AL. Effects of ketamine on major depressive disorder in a patient with posttraumatic stress disorder. *AANA J* 2013;81(2):118–9.

QUESTION SIXTEEN

Robin is a 31-year patient with a history of obsessive compulsive disorder (OCD) being treated with cognitive-behavioral therapy. She is currently 3 months pregnant, and the severity of her obsessions and compulsions have increased during her pregnancy. Which pharmacotherapy would be the preferred option for Robin?

A. Clonazepam

B. Clomipramine

C. Paroxetine

D. Fluoxetine

E. Sertraline

Answer to Question Sixteen

The correct answer is E.

Choice	Peer answers
Clonazepam	2%
Clomipramine	3%
Paroxetine	3%
Fluoxetine	24%
Sertraline	68%

The decision regarding treatment regimen for OCD in women during pregnancy is very difficult. The decision must be based on several factors, such as the risks of untreated maternal psychiatric illness and the known or unknown potential effects of psychotropic medications, benefits of pharmacological treatment, and alternative treatments to medication. Decision-making requires detailed psychiatric assessment including individual and family history of psychiatric disorders, side effects or therapeutic effects of medications, severity of disorder, and degree of impairment in occupational, family, and social areas secondary to the disorder. All steps of the treatment should be administered in agreement with the patient and her relatives. If the patient has severe depression and anxiety symptoms, a high suicide risk, considerable feeding and sleep disturbances secondary to OCD, or has mild to moderate OCD that is unresponsive to cognitive-behavioral therapy, pharmacological treatment regimens may be considered.

A – Incorrect. Clonazepam is generally not effective for OCD. Additionally, exposure to any type of benzodiazepine during the first 3 months of pregnancy should be avoided.

B – Incorrect. In the general population, clomipramine is a first-line agent to treat OCD. However, several studies have suggested an approximately twofold increased risk of cardiovascular defects associated with clomipramine. In addition, the risk of maternal intolerance is relatively high, and the risk for poor neonatal adaptation syndrome (PNAS) is high.

C and D – Incorrect. Paroxetine and fluoxetine are not the best first-line choice because these drugs are the most frequently associated with congenital malformations and PNAS. Data suggest that some birth defects occur 2–3.5 times more frequently among the infants of women treated with paroxetine or fluoxetine early in pregnancy.

E – Correct. A selective serotonin reuptake inhibitor (SSRI) is recommended first-line for the treatment of OCD during pregnancy with adequate risk–benefit assessment. Sertraline is reported to be most effective in OCD, but has the least number of studies focusing on the association with birth defects. The use of pharmacotherapy in moderate to severe OCD must be carefully weighed. As a general rule, the dose of any drug should be as low as possible during pregnancy.

References

Gentile S. Tricyclic antidepressants in pregnancy and puerperium. *Expert Opin Drug Saf* 2014;13:207–25.

Grover S, Avasthi A, Sharma Y. Psychotropics in pregnancy: weighing the risks. *Indian J Med Res* 2006;123(4):497–512.

Goodman JH, Chenausky KL, Freeman MP. Anxiety disorders during pregnancy: a systematic review. *J Clin Psychiatry* 2014;75(10):e1153–84.

Marchesi C, Ossola P, Amerio A, Daniel BD, Tonna M, De Panfilis C. Clinical management of perinatal anxiety disorders: a systematic review. *J Affect Disord* 2016;190:543–50.

Myles N, Newall H, Ward H, Large M. Systematic meta-analysis of individual selective serotonin reuptake inhibitor medications and congenital malformations. *Aust N Z J Psychiatry* 2013;47:1002–12.

Ram D, Gandotra S. Antidepressants, anxiolytics, and hypnotics in pregnancy and lactation. *Indian J Psychiatry* 2015;57(Suppl 2):S354–71.

Reefhuis J, Devine O, Friedman JM, Louik C, Honein MA. Specific SSRIs and birth defects: Bayesian analysis to interpret new data in the context of previous reports. *BMJ* 2015;351:h3190.

Yonkers KA, Wisner KL, Stewart DE, et al. The management of depression during pregnancy: a report from the American Psychiatric Association and the American College of Obstetricians and Gynecologists. *Gen Hosp Psychiatry* 2009;31:403–13.

CHAPTER PEER COMPARISON

For the Anxiety Disorders section, the correct answer was selected 74% of the time.

6 CHRONIC PAIN AND ITS TREATMENT

QUESTION ONE

A 34-year-old woman with fibromyalgia, generalized anxiety disorder, and depression is currently taking several psychotropic medications, including alprazolam, duloxetine, hydrocodone/acetaminophen, and pregabalin. She continues to have residual pain, anxiety, and mood symptoms. Her clinician is considering simplifying her medication regimen and plans to discontinue the medication with the least evidence of efficacy for her disorders. Which of the following should be discontinued?

A. Alprazolam

B. Duloxetine

C. Hydrocodone/acetaminophen

D. Pregabalin

Answer to Question One

The correct answer is C.

Choice	Peer answers
Alprazolam	27%
Duloxetine	2%
Hydrocodone/acetaminophen	67%
Pregabalin	4%

A – Incorrect. Alprazolam is an effective treatment for generalized anxiety disorder.

B – Incorrect. Duloxetine is an effective treatment for both depression and for fibromyalgia.

C – Correct. Hydrocodone/acetaminophen does not have evidence of efficacy for the treatment of fibromyalgia, nor is it an appropriate treatment for his other illnesses.

D – Incorrect. Pregabalin is an effective treatment for fibromyalgia and also has evidence of efficacy in anxiety.

References

Ballantyne JC, Shin NS. Efficacy of opioids for chronic pain: a review of the evidence. *Clin J Pain* 2008;24:469–78.

Clauw DJ. Fibromyalgia: an overview. *Am J Med* 2009;122(Suppl 12):S3–13.

QUESTION TWO

A 35-year-old woman complains of widespread pain so debilitating that she has been unable to work for the last several weeks, although she did not experience any significant injury that seems to account for the pain. Specifically, she states that even the mild pressure of being touched causes such significant pain that she cringes when her two-year-old daughter tries to hug her. This type of pain is called:

A. Acute pain

B. Allodynia

C. Hyperalgesia

D. Neuropathic pain

E. Nociceptive pain

Chronic Pain and its Treatment

Answer to Question Two

The correct answer is B.

Choice	Peer answers
Acute pain	0%
Allodynia	54%
Hyperalgesia	28%
Neuropathic pain	6%
Nociceptive pain	12%

A – Incorrect. Acute pain refers to pain that resolves after a short duration and that is usually directly related to tissue damage. In this case the patient has had significant pain for several weeks despite the lack of any apparent injury; thus, this does not appear to be acute pain.

B – Correct. Allodynia is a painful response to a stimulus that does not normally provoke pain, such as pain in response to light touch. This is consistent with what the patient describes.

C – Incorrect. Hyperalgesia is an exaggerated pain response to something that is normally painful (for example, extreme pain in response to a pin prick). Mild pressure from being hugged by one's child would not normally elicit pain, and thus this particular complaint does not represent hyperalgesia.

D – Incorrect. Neuropathic pain is pain that arises from damage to or dysfunction of any part of the peripheral or central nervous system. Neuropathic pain is not defined by the degree of pain in response to a certain type of stimulus, which is what this patient is describing.

E – Incorrect. Nociceptive pain results from direct activation of pain nerve fibers, either due to chemical, inflammatory, or mechanical mediators, and is usually due to tissue irritation, impending injury, or actual injury. In this case the patient has had significant pain for several weeks despite the lack of any apparent injury; thus, this does not appear to be nociceptive pain.

References
McMahon S, Koltzenburg M (eds). *Wall and Melzack's textbook of pain*, fifth edition. London: Harcourt Publishers; 2005.

Stahl SM. *Stahl's essential psychopharmacology*, fourth edition. New York, NY: Cambridge University Press; 2013. (Chapter 10)

Stahl SM. *Stahl's illustrated chronic pain and fibromyalgia*. New York, NY: Cambridge University Press; 2009. (Chapters 3–4)

Chronic Pain and its Treatment

QUESTION THREE

A young man arrives at the emergency room in great pain after receiving a chemical burn during an accident at work. Which primary afferent neurons would have responded to the chemical stimulus to produce nociceptive neuronal activity?

A. A beta fiber neurons

B. A delta fiber neurons

C. C fiber neurons

Answer to Question Three

The correct answer is C.

Choice	Peer answers
A beta fiber neurons	14%
A delta fiber neurons	35%
C fiber neurons	51%

A – Incorrect. A beta fibers respond to non-noxious small movements such as light touch, hair movement, and vibrations, and do not respond to noxious stimuli.

B – Incorrect. A delta fibers fall somewhere in between A beta fibers and C fiber neurons, sensing noxious mechanical stimuli and subnoxious thermal stimuli.

C – Correct. C fiber peripheral terminals are bare nerve endings that are only activated by noxious mechanical, thermal, or chemical stimuli. Thus C fiber neurons are the primary afferent neurons responsible for nociceptive conduction following this patient's injury.

References

McMahon S, Koltzenburg M (eds). *Wall and Melzack's textbook of pain*, fifth edition. London: Harcourt Publishers; 2005.

Stahl SM. *Stahl's illustrated chronic pain and fibromyalgia*. New York, NY: Cambridge University Press; 2009. (Chapter 2)

Stahl SM. *Stahl's essential psychopharmacology*, fourth edition. New York, NY: Cambridge University Press; 2013. (Chapter 10)

QUESTION FOUR

Fibromyalgia is a syndrome with multiple symptoms that commonly occur together, including widespread pain, decreased pain threshold or tender points, incapacitating fatigue, and anxiety or depression. Which of the following is not part of the current diagnostic criteria for fibromyalgia?

A. A widespread pain index (WPI) score of seven or higher and a symptom severity scale (SS) score of five or higher. Or you have a WPI score of three to six and a SS score of nine or higher

B. Pain has been present for a minimum of 3 months

C. 11 out of 18 points on the body exhibit tenderness

D. There is no other disease that would be causing these symptoms

Chronic Pain and its Treatment

Answer to Question Four

The correct answer is C.

Choice	Peer answers
A widespread pain index (WPI) score of seven or higher and a symptom severity scale (SS) score of five or higher. Or you have a WPI score of three to six and a SS score of nine or higher	27%
Pain has been present for a minimum of 3 months	15%
11 out of 18 points on the body exhibit tenderness	51%
There is no other disease that would be causing these symptoms	6%

A – Incorrect. The widespread pain index (WPI) and symptom severity scale (SS) are used to check for signs of fibromyalgia.

B – Incorrect. To be diagnosed with fibromyalgia, patients need to have experienced symptoms at a similar level for at least 3 months.

C – Correct. The official diagnostic criteria for fibromyalgia no longer require a tender point examination. The tender point criteria, which are part of the 1990 American College of Rheumatology (ACR) criteria for fibromyalgia, required tenderness on pressure (tender points) in at least 11 of 18 specified sites and the presence of widespread pain for diagnosis. Over time, experts have realized that many doctors didn't know how to check for tender points or refused to do so. Plus, the older system didn't account for many symptoms that have since been recognized as key features of fibromyalgia (e.g., fatigue or depression).

D – Incorrect. Many conditions can cause symptoms similar to those of fibromyalgia. Providers must rule out those conditions to make an accurate diagnosis.

References

Bennett RM, Friend R, Marcus D, et al. Criteria for the diagnosis of fibromyalgia: validation of the modified 2010 preliminary American College of Rheumatology criteria and the development of alternative criteria. *Arthritis Care Res (Hoboken)* 2014;66(9):1364–73.

Wolfe F, Clauw DJ, Fitzcharles MA, et al. The American College of Rheumatology preliminary diagnostic criteria for fibromyalgia and measurement of symptom severity. *Arthritis Care Res (Hoboken)* 2010;62(5):600–10.

QUESTION FIVE

A 29-year-old woman has just been diagnosed with major depressive disorder and is being prescribed a selective serotonin reuptake inhibitor (SSRI). In addition to depressed mood, lack of interest in her work or friends, and difficulty sleeping, she has been experiencing aches and pains in her arms, shoulders, and torso. She asks if the SSRI is likely to alleviate her painful physical symptoms as well as her emotional ones. Which of the following statements is true?

A. SSRIs may have inconsistent effects on pain because serotonin can both inhibit and facilitate ascending nociceptive signals

B. SSRIs may worsen pain because serotonin can facilitate but not inhibit ascending nociceptive signals

C. SSRIs generally alleviate pain because serotonin can inhibit but not facilitate ascending nociceptive signals

D. SSRIs generally have no effect on pain because serotonin neither facilitates nor inhibits nociceptive signals

Answer to Question Five

The correct answer is A.

Choice	Peer answers
SSRIs may have inconsistent effects on pain because serotonin can both inhibit and facilitate ascending nociceptive signals	64%
SSRIs may worsen pain because serotonin can facilitate but not inhibit ascending nociceptive signals	0%
SSRIs generally alleviate pain because serotonin can inhibit but not facilitate ascending nociceptive signals	18%
SSRIs generally have no effect on pain because serotonin neither facilitates nor inhibits nociceptive signals	18%

Two important descending pathways that inhibit ascending nociceptive signals are the noradrenergic and the serotonergic pathways. Thus, enhancement of neurotransmission in either of these pathways could contribute to alleviation of chronic pain.

However, serotonin is also a major neurotransmitter in descending facilitation pathways to the spinal cord. The combination of both inhibitory and facilitatory actions of serotonin may explain why SSRIs seem to have inconsistent effects on painful somatic symptoms.

A – Correct. (SSRIs may have inconsistent effects on pain because serotonin can both inhibit and facilitate ascending nociceptive signals.)

B – Incorrect. (SSRIs may worsen pain because serotonin can facilitate but not inhibit ascending nociceptive signals.)

C – Incorrect. (SSRIs generally alleviate pain because serotonin can inhibit but not facilitate ascending nociceptive signals.)

D – Incorrect. (SSRIs generally have no effect on pain because serotonin neither facilitates nor inhibits nociceptive signals.)

References
Stahl SM. *Stahl's illustrated chronic pain and fibromyalgia*. New York, NY: Cambridge University Press; 2009. (Chapter 5)
Stahl SM. *Stahl's essential psychopharmacology, fourth edition*. New York, NY: Cambridge University Press; 2013. (Chapter 10)

QUESTION SIX

A 22-year-old woman with pain throughout her body, extreme fatigue, and poor sleep is diagnosed with fibromyalgia. Her care provider considers prescribing pregabalin, which may alleviate pain by:

A. Binding to the closed conformation of voltage-sensitive sodium channels

B. Binding to the open conformation of voltage-sensitive sodium channels

C. Binding to the closed conformation of voltage-sensitive calcium channels

D. Binding to the open conformation of voltage-sensitive calcium channels

Chronic Pain and its Treatment

Answer to Question Six

The correct answer is D.

Choice	Peer answers
Binding to the closed conformation of voltage-sensitive sodium channels	8%
Binding to the open conformation of voltage-sensitive sodium channels	21%
Binding to the closed conformation of voltage-sensitive calcium channels	14%
Binding to the open conformation of voltage-sensitive calcium channels	56%

A and B – Incorrect. Both voltage-sensitive sodium and voltage-sensitive calcium channels (VSCCs) are involved in transmission of pain; however, pregabalin does not bind to voltage-sensitive sodium channels in any conformation.

C – Incorrect. This molecular action predicts more affinity for VSCCs that are actively conducting neuronal impulses within the pain pathway and thus a selective action on those VSCCs causing neuropathic pain, ignoring other VSCCs that are closed, and thus not interfering with normal neurotransmission in central neurons uninvolved in mediating the pathological pain state.

D – Correct. Pregabalin does, however, bind to the alpha 2 delta subunit of VSCCs. In fact, pregabalin binds preferentially to the open conformation of these channels and thus may be particularly effective in blocking channels that are the most active, with a "use-dependent" form of inhibition.

References
Dooley DJ, Taylor CP, Donevan S, Feltner D. Ca2+ channel alpha 2 delta ligands: novel modulators of neurotransmission. *Trends Pharmacol Sci* 2007;28:75–82.

Stahl SM. *Stahl's illustrated chronic pain and fibromyalgia*. New York, NY: Cambridge University Press; 2009. (Chapter 5)

Stahl SM. *Stahl's essential psychopharmacology*, fourth edition. New York, NY: Cambridge University Press; 2013. (Chapter 10)

QUESTION SEVEN

A 30-year-old man with juvenile-onset diabetes has begun experiencing throbbing pain, particularly at night. In addition, he states that his body generally feels sensitive all over, so that even the brush of his clothes against his skin can be uncomfortable. These symptoms, indicative of diabetic peripheral neuropathy, may be caused by:

A. Inflammation or damage in the periphery without disturbance in central pain processing

B. Central disturbance in pain processing without damage in the periphery

C. Inflammation or damage in the periphery combined with central disturbance in pain processing

Answer to Question Seven

The correct answer is C.

Choice	Peer answers
Inflammation or damage in the periphery without disturbance in central pain processing	19%
Central disturbance in pain processing without damage in the periphery	3%
Inflammation or damage in the periphery combined with central disturbance in pain processing	78%

A and B – Incorrect.

C – Correct. Chronic pain syndromes may be peripheral, central, or both peripheral and central ("mixed") in origin. Over time, diabetes can cause inflammation that damages peripheral nerves and thus leads to painful physical symptoms. In addition, that damage may cause repetitive activation of nociception, and such ongoing neuronal activity may induce central plasticity within the pain pathway, with progressive and potentially irreversible molecular changes in pain processing pathways eventually leading to progressive and potentially irreversible pain symptoms. Thus, diabetic peripheral neuropathy is a syndrome in which definite peripheral injury is combined with central sensitization.

References

Stahl SM. *Stahl's illustrated chronic pain and fibromyalgia*. New York, NY: Cambridge University Press; 2009. (Chapter 2)

Stahl SM. *Stahl's essential psychopharmacology*, fourth edition. New York, NY: Cambridge University Press; 2013. (Chapter 10)

QUESTION EIGHT

A 34-year-old man presents with chronic back pain and a major depressive episode. Which of the following are documented to treat both chronic central pain and depression without significant side effects?

A. Amitriptyline

B. Duloxetine

C. Gabapentin

D. Sertaline

Answer to Question Eight

The correct answer is B.

Choice	Peer answers
Amitriptyline	6%
Duloxetine	92%
Gabapentin	1%
Sertaline	1%

A – Incorrect. Although effective for depression and chronic pain, tricyclics antidepressants (TCAs) like amitriptyline have several unwanted mechanisms. Histamine 1 receptor blockade causes sedation and may lead to weight gain. Muscarinic M1 receptor blockade causes dry mouth, blurred vision, urinary retention, and constipation; and muscarinic M3 receptor blockade can interfere with insulin action. Alpha 1 adrenergic receptor blockade causes orthostatic hypotension and dizziness.

B – Correct. Duloxetine, a serotonin norepinephrine reuptake inhibitor, may be the antidepressant that is best documented to have efficacy in pain conditions. Duloxetine targets both descending noradrenergic and serotonergic projections and the patient may benefit from an antidepressant with dual mechanisms, which may help alleviate her chronic pain.

C – Incorrect. Gabapentin, an alpha 2 delta ligand, is not documented to show efficacy in the treatment of depression.

D – Incorrect. Sertraline, a selective serotonin reuptake inhibitor, is not documented to treat chronic central pain. It is also possible that the patient may benefit instead from an antidepressant treatment with dual mechanisms, particularly one with noradrenergic properties, which may help alleviate her chronic pain.

References

Stahl SM. *Stahl's essential psychopharmacology*, fourth edition. New York, NY: Cambridge University Press; 2013. (Chapter 10)

Stahl SM. *Stahl's essential psychopharmacology: the prescriber's guide*, sixth edition. New York, NY: Cambridge University Press; 2017.

Chronic Pain and its Treatment

QUESTION NINE

A 36-year-old woman has just been diagnosed with fibromyalgia. In addition to her painful physical symptoms, she is experiencing problems with memory and significant difficulty concentrating at work. Which of the following may be most likely to alleviate both her physical pain and her cognitive symptoms?

A. Bupropion

B. Cyclobenzaprine

C. Milnacipran

D. Pregabalin

Answer to Question Nine

The correct answer is C.

Choice	Peer answers
Bupropion	28%
Cyclobenzaprine	3%
Milnacipran	55%
Pregabalin	15%

Documented mechanisms for alleviating central neuropathic pain include enhancement of serotonergic and noradrenergic neurotransmission in descending spinal pathways as well as reduction of calcium influx in pain pathways. Cognitive dysfunction may be alleviated by increasing dopaminergic (and possibly noradrenergic) neurotransmission in the dorsolateral prefrontal cortex.

A – Incorrect. Bupropion is a norepinephrine and dopamine reuptake inhibitor (NDRI) and may reduce cognitive symptoms associated with fibromyalgia when used as adjunct, but is not documented to reduce pain.

B – Incorrect. Cyclobenzaprine is a muscle relaxant and may be used for fibromyalgia, but is not generally a first-line choice and does not have efficacy for cognitive symptoms.

C – Correct. Milnacipran is a serotonin and norepinephrine reuptake inhibitor (SNRI) with documented efficacy for treating neuro-pathic pain. In addition, it can also improve cognitive symptoms through its potent norepinephrine reuptake binding property.

D – Incorrect. Pregabalin binds to the alpha 2 delta subunit of volt-age-sensitive calcium channels to reduce calcium influx. It has documented efficacy for treating neuropathic pain, but is not docu-mented to reduce cognitive symptoms.

References

Stahl SM. *Case studies: Stahl's essential psychopharmacology.* New York, NY: Cambridge University Press; 2011.

Stahl SM. *Stahl's essential psychopharmacology*, fourth edition. New York, NY: Cambridge University Press; 2013. (Chapter 10)

QUESTION TEN

A 44-year-old male patient with chronic hepatitis is seeking treatment for chronic neuropathic pain. Which of the following would you most likely avoid prescribing for this patient?

A. Duloxetine

B. Gabapentin

C. Pregabalin

Answer to Question Ten

The correct answer is A.

Choice	Peer answers
Duloxetine	76%
Gabapentin	14%
Pregabalin	10%

All of these medications can be effective for chronic neuropathic pain; what distinguishes them here is their effects in hepatic impairment.

A – Correct. Duloxetine increases the risk of elevation of serum transaminase levels and is not recommended for use in individuals with hepatic insufficiency; thus it would not be recommended in this case.

B and C – Incorrect. Gabapentin and pregabalin are not metabolized by the liver, nor do they appear to have effects on liver functioning; thus they are considered safe in hepatic impairment and do not generally require dose adjustment.

References

Scholz BA, Hammonds CL, Boomershine CS. Duloxetine for the management of fibromyalgia syndrome. *J Pain Res* 2009;2:99–108.

Stahl SM. *Stahl's essential psychopharmacology: the prescriber's guide*, sixth edition. New York, NY: Cambridge University Press; 2017.

QUESTION ELEVEN

A 28-year-old patient with a long history of painful somatic symptoms has been diagnosed with major depressive disorder but has not responded to multiple successive trials of selective serotonin reuptake inhibitors (SSRIs). Her clinician is now considering prescribing a monoamine oxidase inhibitor (MAOI). Due to her history of chronic pain, she is currently taking an opioid. Which of the following opioids would be of greatest concern for this patient?

A. Codeine

B. Morphine

C. Hydrocodone

D. Meperidine

Chronic Pain and its Treatment

Answer to Question Eleven

The correct answer is D.

Choice	Peer answers
Codeine	3%
Morphine	12%
Hydrocodone	9%
Meperidine	77%

There is no interaction of MAOIs with opioid mechanisms; however, some opioids have serotonergic properties that could increase risk of serotonin syndrome if they were administered together.

A – Incorrect. Codeine does not have serotonergic properties and is safe to prescribe with MAOIs.

B – Incorrect. Morphine does not have serotonergic properties and is safe to prescribe with MAOIs.

C – Incorrect. Hydrocodone does not have serotonergic properties and is safe to prescribe with MAOIs.

D – Correct. Meperidine is a potent serotonin reuptake inhibitor and should not be prescribed with MAOIs.

References
Stahl SM, Felker A. Monoamine oxidase inhibitors: a modern guide to an unrequited class of antidepressants. *CNS Spectr* 2008;13(10):855–70.

Wimbiscus M, Kostenko O, Malone D. MAO inhibitors: risks, benefits, and lore. *Curr Drug Therapy* 2010;77(2):859–82.

QUESTION TWELVE

Your patient, a 33-year-old woman whom you have been treating for 3 years for major depressive disorder, discloses to you that 6 weeks ago, she visited a cannabis clinic and was certified for the use of medical marijuana to treat chronic back pain resulting from a car accident and subsequent surgery 2 years ago. Recent systematic reviews have suggested cannabinoids demonstrate a modest effect on chronic pain. Which of the following statements is true about the cannabinoid receptor regarding pain?

A. Activation of cannabinoid receptor 1 (CB1), found in high concentration on immune cells, may decrease inflammation

B. Activation of cannabinoid receptor 2 (CB2) receptors, found in high concentrations in areas of the central nervous system (CNS), may control pain perception

C. Activation of cannabinoid receptor 1 (CB1), found in high concentration on neuron terminals, may decrease inflammation

D. Activation of cannabinoid receptor 2 (CB2) receptors on immune cells may decrease inflammation and nociceptor excitation, reducing pain sensitivity

Chronic Pain and its Treatment

Answer to Question Twelve

The correct answer is D.

Choice	Peer answers
Activation of cannabinoid receptor 1 (CB1), found in high concentration on immune cells, may decrease inflammation	3%
Activation of cannabinoid receptor 2 (CB2) receptors, found in high concentrations in areas of the central nervous system (CNS), may control pain perception	32%
Activation of cannabinoid receptor 1 (CB1), found in high concentration on neuron terminals, may decrease inflammation	13%
Activation of cannabinoid receptor 2 (CB2) receptors on immune cells may decrease inflammation and nociceptor excitation, reducing pain sensitivity	53%

A – Incorrect. CB1 receptors are found in high concentrations on terminals of central and peripheral neurons. Activation of CB1 receptors found on peripheral neuron terminals of primary sensory neurons may inhibit pain transmission.

B – Incorrect. CB2 receptors are predominantly found in the immune system, or on immune-derived cells with the greatest density in the spleen and are not found in high concentration in the CNS.

C – Incorrect. CB1 receptors are found in high concentrations on terminals of central and peripheral neurons. Activation of CB1 receptors found on peripheral neuron terminals of primary sensory neurons may inhibit pain transmission. CB2 receptors found on immune cells may decrease inflammation.

D – Correct. CB2 receptors are predominantly found in the immune system, or on immune-derived cells with the greatest density in the spleen. Additionally, recent studies suggest that CB2 receptors are also present in the CNS. CB2 receptors are thought to serve an important role in immune function and inflammation. There is evidence that CB2 receptor activation reduces nociception in a variety of preclinical models, including those involving tactile and thermal allodynia, mechanical and thermal hyperalgesia, and writhing.

Reference

Abrams DI, Couey P, Shade SB, Kelly ME, Benowitz NL. Cannabinoid–opioid interaction in chronic pain. *Clin Pharmacol Ther* 2011;90(6):844–51.

Andreae MH, Carter GM, Shaparin N, et al. Inhaled cannabis for chronic neuropathic pain: a meta-analysis of individual patient data. *J Pain* 2015;16(12):1221–32.

Beltramo M. Cannabinoid type 2 receptor as a target for chronic pain. *Mini Rev Med Chem* 2009;9(1):11–25.

National Academies of Sciences, Engineering, and Medicine. *The Health Effects of Cannabis and Cannabinoids: The Current State of Evidence and Recommendations for Research.* Washington, DC: The National Academies Press; 2017. doi:https://doi.org/10.17226/24625.

Walker JM, Hohmann AG, Martin WJ, Strangman NM, Huang SM, Tsou K. The neurobiology of cannabinoid analgesia. *Life Sci* 1999;65(6–7):665–73.

Whiting PF, Wolff RF, Deshpande S et al. Cannabinoids for medical use: a systematic review and meta-analysis. *JAMA* 2015;313(24): 2456–73.

CHAPTER PEER COMPARISON

For the Chronic Pain section, the correct answer was selected 64% of the time.

7 DISORDERS OF SLEEP AND WAKEFULNESS AND THEIR TREATMENT

QUESTION ONE

Denise is a 32–year–old patient with shift work disorder who reports that she is having difficulty in her job as a pastry chef due to excessive sleepiness during her shift. Which of the following is a potential therapeutic mechanism to promote wakefulness?

A. Inhibit GABA activity

B. Inhibit histamine activity

C. Inhibit orexin activity

D. All of the above

E. None of the above

Answer to Question One

The correct answer is A.

Choice	Peer answers
Inhibit GABA activity	53%
Inhibit histamine activity	5%
Inhibit orexin activity	8%
All of the above	30%
None of the above	5%

The hypothalamus is a key control center for sleep and wake, and the specific circuitry that regulates sleep/wake is called the sleep/wake switch. The "off" setting, or sleep promoter, is localized within the ventrolateral preoptic nucleus (VLPO) of the hypothalamus, while "on" – the wake promoter – is localized within the tuberomammillary nucleus (TMN) of the hypothalamus. Two key neurotransmitters regulate the sleep/wake switch: histamine from the TMN and GABA from the VLPO.

A – Correct. When the VLPO is active and GABA is released to the TMN, the sleep promoter is on and the wake promoter is inhibited. Thus, inhibiting GABA activity can promote wakefulness.

B – Incorrect. When the TMN is active and histamine is released to the cortex and the VLPO, the wake promoter is on and the sleep promoter is inhibited. Thus, inhibiting histamine activity can promote sleep, not wakefulness.

C – Incorrect. The sleep/wake switch is also regulated by orexin neurons in the lateral hypothalamus, which stabilize wakefulness. Inhibition of orexin would therefore promote sleep, not wakefulness. In fact, a deficiency of orexin is an underlying cause of the extreme and sudden sleepiness seen in narcolepsy.

References
Stahl SM. *Stahl's essential psychopharmacology*, fourth edition. New York, NY: Cambridge University Press; 2013. (Chapter 11)

Stahl SM, Morrissette DA. *Stahl's illustrated sleep and wake disorders*. Cambridge: Cambridge University Press; 2016.

QUESTION TWO

A 72-year-old woman has been having difficulty sleeping for several weeks, including both difficulty falling asleep and frequent nighttime awakenings. Medical examination rules out an underlying condition contributing to insomnia, and she is not taking any medications that are associated with disrupted sleep. The patient is retired and spends the day caring for her grandchildren, including driving the older ones to school in the morning. Which of the following would be the most appropriate treatment option for this patient?

A. Flurazepam

B. Temazepam

C. Zaleplon

D. Zolpidem CR

Answer to Question Two

The correct answer is D.

Choice	Peer answers
Flurazepam	1%
Temazepam	12%
Zaleplon	28%
Zolpidem CR	59%

The half-lives of hypnotics can have an important impact on their tolerability and efficacy profiles.

A – Incorrect. Hypnotics with ultra-long half-lives (greater than 24 hours: for example, flurazepam and quazepam) can cause drug accumulation with chronic use. This can cause impairment that has been associated with increased risk of falls, particularly in the elderly.

B – Incorrect. Hypnotics with moderate half-lives (15–30 hours: estazolam, temazepam, most tricyclic antidepressants, mirtazapine, olanzapine) may not wear off until after the individual needs to awaken and thus may have "hangover" effects (sedation, memory problems). Given that the patient needs to drive early in the morning, this may not be the best option for her.

C – Incorrect. Hypnotics with ultra-short half-lives (1–3 hours: zaleplon, triazolam, zolpidem, melatonin, ramelteon) can wear off before the individual needs to awaken and thus cause loss of sleep maintenance, which is already a problem for this patient.

D – Correct. Hypnotics with half-lives that are short but not ultra-short (approximately 6 hours: zolpidem CR, eszopiclone, and perhaps low doses of trazodone or doxepin) may provide rapid onset of action and plasma levels above the minimally effective concentration only for the duration of a normal night's sleep. Thus, of the answer choices, zolpidem CR may best treat the patient's difficulties with sleep onset and maintenance while avoiding risks associated with agents with longer half-lives. The dose of zolpidem CR in elderly patients is 6.25 mg/night.

References

Stahl SM. *Stahl's essential psychopharmacology*, fourth edition. New York, NY: Cambridge University Press; 2013. (Chapter 11)

Stahl SM. *Stahl's essential psychopharmacology, the prescriber's guide*, sixth edition. New York, NY: Cambridge University Press; 2017.

QUESTION THREE

A 75-year-old man in good physical shape is having sleep problems. He wakes up at 4 a.m. and although he tries to stay awake in the evening to prevent this early rising, he usually falls asleep right after dinner, often before 7 p.m. Which of the following treatment options may be most beneficial for this patient?

A. Early morning melatonin

B. Evening melatonin

C. Late afternoon/evening light

D. A and C

E. A and B

F. B and C

Answer to Question Three

The correct answer is D.

Choice	Peer answers
Early morning melatonin	2%
Evening melatonin	3%
Late afternoon/evening light	18%
A and C	51%
A and B	0%
B and C	24%

A and C – Partially correct.

B, E, and F – Incorrect. Evening melatonin would not be appropriate for this patient who is phase-advanced. Rather, evening melatonin (and morning light) may benefit patients with phase-delayed circadian rhythms, potentially resetting the suprachiasmatic nucleus (SCN) so that the sleep/wake switch turns on earlier.

D – Correct. This patient is phase-advanced. Phase-advanced circadian rhythms may benefit from early morning melatonin and evening light, which could help reset the SCN so that the sleep/wake switch stays off longer.

References

Dodson ER, Zee PC. Therapeutics for circadian rhythm sleep disorders. *Sleep Med Clin* 2010;5(4):701–15.

Edwards BA, O'Driscoll DM, Ali A, Jordon AS, Trinder J, Malhotra A. Aging and sleep: physiology and pathophysiology. *Semin Respir Crit Care Med* 2010;31(5):618–33.

Stahl SM. *Case studies: Stahl's essential psychopharmacology*. New York, NY: Cambridge University Press; 2011.

QUESTION FOUR

A 45-year-old woman was prescribed doxepin 10 mg/night for insomnia. She reports that it helped only a little, so she has been increasing the dose, up to 100 mg/night, as an attempt to increase the hypnotic effects (with some success). She also reports dizzy spells and constipation. Which property does doxepin exhibit in higher doses that could be the cause of these side effects?

A. Inhibiting reuptake of serotonin and norepinephrine

B. 5HT2A and 5HT2C antagonism

C. Alpha 1 adrenergic and muscarinic 1 antagonism

D. 5HT2A and 5HT2B antagonism

Disorders of Sleep and Wakefulness and their Treatment

Answer to Question Four

The correct answer is C.

Choice	Peer answers
Inhibiting reuptake of serotonin and norepinephrine	3%
5HT2A and 5HT2C antagonism	5%
Alpha 1 adrenergic and muscarinic 1 antagonism	90%
5HT2A and 5HT2B antagonism	1%

A, B, and D – Incorrect. Higher doses of doxepin inhibit reuptake of serotonin and norepinephrine, but such effects are not likely to explain these side effects.

C – Correct. Low-dose doxepin is selective for histamine 1 receptors, which is why it can act as a hypnotic. It is likely that alpha 1 adrenergic and muscarinic 1 receptor antagonism seen with higher doses of doxepin would explain these side effects.

References

Stahl SM. Selective histamine H1 antagonism: novel hypnotic and pharmacologic actions challenge classical notions of antihistamines. *CNS Spectr* 2008;13(12):1027–38.

Stahl SM. *Stahl's essential psychopharmacology*, fourth edition. New York, NY: Cambridge University Press; 2013. (Chapter 11)

Stahl SM. *Stahl's essential psychopharmacology, the prescriber's guide*, sixth edition. New York, NY: Cambridge University Press; 2017.

QUESTION FIVE

Although he sleeps soundly through the night, a 54-year-old man, whom you have previously treated for depression, describes feeling physically exhausted, sometimes with sore muscles, when he wakes up in the morning. His wife reports that she frequently wakes in the middle of the night from his movements. Which of the following tests would you refer him to take?

A. Polysomnograph

B. Multiple sleep latency test

C. Maintenance of wakefulness test

D. A, B, and C

Disorders of Sleep and Wakefulness and their Treatment

Answer to Question Five

The correct answer is A.

Choice	Peer answers
Polysomnograph	73%
Multiple sleep latency test	4%
Maintenance of wakefulness test	1%
A, B, and C	22%

A – Correct. It is likely that this patient is suffering from periodic limb movements of sleep (PLMS) or periodic limb movement disorder (PLMD), for which a polysomnograph test is recommended.

B – Incorrect. Multiple sleep latency tests are recommended for narcolepsy without cataplexy and idiopathic hypersomnia.

C – Incorrect. Maintenance of wakefulness tests are recommended for treatment assessment for narcolepsy, with or without cataplexy and idiopathic hypersomnia.

D – Incorrect.

References

Kushida CA, **Littner MR**, **Morgenthaler T** et al. Practice parameters for the indications for polysomnography and related procedures: an update for 2005. *Sleep* 2005;28(4):499–521.

Littner MR, **Kushida CA**, **Wise M** et al. Practice parameters for clinical use of the multiple sleep latency test and the maintenance of wakefulness test. *Sleep* 2005;28(1):113–21.

QUESTION SIX

A patient started working a night shift as a security guard 1 week ago. At this time, he is most likely to have a disrupted _____ drive while his _____ drive is unaffected.

A. Ultradian ... circadian

B. Circadian ... homeostatic

C. Homeostatic ... ultradian

D. Ultradian ... homeostatic

E. Circadian ... ultradian

F. Homeostatic ... circadian

Answer to Question Six

The correct answer is B.

Choice	Peer answers
Ultradian ... circadian	6%
Circadian ... homeostatic	64%
Homeostatic ... ultradian	0%
Ultradian ... homeostatic	1%
Circadian ... ultradian	21%
Homeostatic ... circadian	8%

A, C, D, and E – Incorrect. Ultradian cycle refers to the cyclical recurrence of the multiple phases of sleep and is most likely unaffected in this normal individual.

B – Correct. Circadian (wake) drive is the result of input such as light, melatonin, and physical activity to the suprachiasmatic nucleus. Homeostatic (sleep) drive increases the longer one is awake without sleep and is associated with an accumulation of the neurotransmitter adenosine. An individual working a night shift is not likely to receive normal light input although (s)he may sleep a normal amount and therefore is likely to have a disrupted circadian drive with an unaffected homeostatic drive.

Over time, however, individuals who do shift work often sleep fewer hours than they would on a normal schedule – but not because they actually need less sleep – and thus their homeostatic drive can build up.

F – Incorrect.

References

Czeisler CA, Gooley JJ. Sleep and circadian rhythms in humans. *Cold Spring Harb Symp Quant Biol* 2007;72:579–97.

Stahl SM. *Stahl's essential psychopharmacology*, fourth edition. New York, NY: Cambridge University Press; 2013. (Chapter 11)

QUESTION SEVEN

A clinician is planning to prescribe eszopiclone for a 34-year-old male patient with insomnia. What is the correct starting dose for this patient?

A. 0.5 mg/night

B. 1 mg/night

C. 2 mg/night

D. 3 mg/night

Answer to Question Seven

The correct answer is B.

Choice	Peer answers
0.5 mg/night	19%
1 mg/night	67%
2 mg/night	11%
3 mg/night	3%

A – Incorrect (0.5 mg/night).

B – Correct. In 2014 the FDA reduced the recommended starting dose of eszopiclone from 2 mg/night to 1 mg/night for both men and women. This is because, in some patients, eszopiclone blood levels may be high enough the next morning to cause impairment in activities that require alertness, including driving. In 2013, the FDA issued new dosing requirements for zolpidem due to the risk of next-morning impairment. However, the label change applied only to dosing in women (5 mg IR, 6.25 mg XR).

C – Incorrect (2 mg/night). Prior to the revised dosing requirements in 2014, the recommended dose range for eszopiclone was 2–3 mg/night; however, that is no longer the case.

D – Incorrect (3 mg/night). Prior to the revised dosing requirements in 2014, the recommended dose range for eszopiclone was 2–3 mg/night; however, that is no longer the case.

References
Stahl SM. *Stahl's essential psychopharmacology, the prescriber's guide*, sixth edition. New York, NY: Cambridge University Press; 2017.

QUESTION EIGHT

A 28-year-old woman with chronic insomnia is hoping to find an effective treatment but is reluctant to try anything that might cause dependence. Her clinician is considering prescribing suvorexant, which acts as an antagonist at orexin receptors. Specifically, what type of orexin antagonists may be effective for treating patients with sleep–wake disorders?

A. Single orexin receptor antagonists selective for orexin 1 receptors

B. Single orexin receptor antagonists selective for orexin 2 receptors

C. Dual orexin receptor antagonists that block both orexin 1 and 2 receptors

D. A and B

E. B and C

Answer to Question Eight

The correct answer is E.

Choice	Peer answers
Single orexin receptor antagonists selective for orexin 1 receptors	15%
Single orexin receptor antagonists selective for orexin 2 receptors	12%
Dual orexin receptor antagonists that block both orexin 1 and 2 receptors	37%
A and B	6%
B and C	31%

A – Incorrect. Orexin serves to stabilize and promote wakefulness. Its postsynaptic actions are mediated by two receptors: orexin 1 and orexin 2. Orexin 1 receptors are highly expressed in the locus coeruleus, where noradrenergic neurons originate, and are thought to play only a supplementary role in sleep/wake regulation. Consistent with this, preclinical trials with single orexin receptor antagonists for orexin 1 receptors have not demonstrated an effect on sleep.

B – Partially correct. Orexin 2 receptors are highly expressed in the tuberomammillary nucleus, where histaminergic neurons originate. It is believed that the effect of orexin on wakefulness is largely mediated by activation of the TMN histaminergic neurons that express orexin 2 receptors. Presumably, orexin 2 receptors therefore play a pivotal role in sleep/wake regulation. Consistent with this, there are promising preclinical results of single orexin receptor antagonists for orexin 2 receptors.

C – Partially correct. Dual orexin receptor antagonists, such as suvorexant, have evidence of efficacy in the treatment of insomnia.

D – Incorrect (A and B).

E – Correct (B and C).

References

Stahl SM. *Stahl's essential psychopharmacology*, fourth edition. New York, NY: Cambridge University Press; 2013.

QUESTION NINE

The suprachiasmatic nucleus, or "circadian pacemaker," is influenced by activity, light, and which one of the following neurotransmitters?

A. Acetylcholine

B. Melatonin

C. Norepinephrine

D. Serotonin

Answer to Question Nine

The correct answer is B.

Choice	Peer answers
Acetylcholine	3%
Melatonin	94%
Norepinephrine	0%
Serotonin	2%

A – Incorrect. Acetylcholine is formed in cholinergic neurons and is primarily involved in cognitive functioning. It does not have a prominent role in regulation of circadian rhythms.

B – Correct. Melatonin is secreted by the pineal gland and mainly acts in the suprachiasmatic nucleus to regulate circadian rhythms.

C – Incorrect. Norepinephrine is involved in many functions, including sleep. However, it does not have a primary role in regulating the suprachiasmatic nucleus.

D – Incorrect. Serotonin, like norepinephrine, is involved in many functions, including sleep. It does not, however, play a prominent role in regulating the suprachiasmatic nucleus.

References

Arendt J. Melatonin and the pineal gland: influence on mammalian seasonal and circadian physiology. *Rev Reproduction* 1998;3:13–22.

Stahl SM. *Stahl's essential psychopharmacology*, fourth edition. New York, NY: Cambridge University Press; 2013. (Chapter 11)

Stahl SM, Morrissette DA. *Stahl's illustrated sleep and wake disorders*. Cambridge: Cambridge University Press; 2016.

QUESTION TEN

Rachel is an obese 35-year-old woman who works the night shift as an emergency medical responder. Recent evidence indicates that a disrupted sleep/wake cycle may increase one's risk for obesity, diabetes, and cardiovascular disease by:

A. Increasing levels of leptin

B. Increasing levels of ghrelin

C. Increasing levels of both leptin and ghrelin

D. Decreasing levels of both leptin and ghrelin

Answer to Question Ten

The correct answer is B.

Choice	Peer answers
Increasing levels of leptin	10%
Increasing levels of ghrelin	38%
Increasing levels of both leptin and ghrelin	44%
Decreasing levels of both leptin and ghrelin	8%

A – Incorrect. Leptin is an anorectic (appetite-inhibiting) hormone. Increasing levels of leptin would therefore be expected to cause weight loss rather than obesity. Indeed, a disrupted sleep/wake cycle has been shown to decrease levels of leptin.

B – Correct. Ghrelin is an orexigenic (appetite-stimulating) hormone. A disrupted sleep/wake cycle has been shown to increase levels of ghrelin; this increase in ghrelin is hypothesized to contribute to the increased risk of obesity, diabetes, and cardiovascular disease.

C and D – Incorrect. A disrupted sleep/wake cycle has been shown to decrease circulating levels of the anorectic (appetite-inhibiting) hormone leptin and increase circulating levels of the orexigenic (appetite-stimulating) hormone ghrelin.

References
Froy O. Metabolism and circadian rhythms – implications for obesity. *Endocr Rev* 2010;31(1):1–24.

Golombek DA, **Casiraghi LP**, **Agostino PV**, et al. The times they are a-changing: effects of circadian desynchronization on physiology and disease. *J Physiol Paris* 2013;107:310–22.

Nixon JP, **Mavanji V**, **Butterick TA**, et al. Sleep disorders, obesity, and aging: the role of orexin. *Aging Res Rev* 2015;20:63–73.

Orzel-Gryglewska J. Consequences of sleep deprivation. *Int J Occup Med Environ Health* 2010;23(1):95–114.

Stahl SM, **Morrissette DA**. *Stahl's illustrated sleep and wake disorders.* Cambridge: Cambridge University Press; 2016.

QUESTION ELEVEN

A 12-year-old male patient has been brought to the clinic by his parents for evaluation. The patient typically sleeps for 10 or more hours a day (yet still exhibits excessive daytime sleepiness), eats excessive amounts of food, and demonstrates disinhibited behaviors including masturbation in public places. This patient most likely has:

A. Idiopathic hypersomnia

B. Narcolepsy without cataplexy

C. Kleine–Levin syndrome

Answer to Question Eleven

The correct answer is C.

Choice	Peer answers
A. Idiopathic hypersomnia	2%
B. Narcolepsy without cataplexy	4%
Kleine–Levin syndrome	94%

A – Incorrect. Idiopathic hypersomnia is characterized by either long or normal sleep duration accompanied by constant excessive daytime sleepiness, short sleep onset latency, and complaints of non-refreshing sleep. Patients with idiopathic hypersomnia may also report sleep drunkenness and somnolence following sleep. The diagnosis of idiopathic hypersomnia includes excessive daytime sleepiness lasting at least 3 months; a sleep latency of under 8 minutes, as determined by the Multiple Sleep Latency Test (MSLT); and fewer than 2 sleep onset REM periods (SOREMPs). Although some of the symptoms that this patient is experiencing, including excessive daytime sleepiness despite long sleep duration, are in line with idiopathic hypersomnia, the additional symptoms being exhibited by this patient (including disinhibited and compulsive behaviors) are suggestive of Kleine–Levin syndrome.

B – Incorrect. Narcolepsy is characterized by excessive daytime sleepiness, the intrusion of sleep during periods of wakefulness, and abnormal REM sleep, including periods of REM occurring at the onset of sleep (SOREMPs). Although some of the symptoms that this patient is experiencing, including excessive daytime sleepiness, are in line with idiopathic hypersomnia, the additional symptoms being exhibited by this patient (including disinhibited and compulsive behaviors) are suggestive of Kleine–Levin syndrome.

C – Correct. Kleine–Levin syndrome is the most common form of recurrent hypersomnia. This rare disorder mostly affects adolescent boys and is characterized by bouts of hypersomnolence coupled with cognitive and mood disturbances, compulsive eating, hypersexuality, and disinhibited behavior.

References
Adenuga O, Attarian H. Treatment of disorders of hypersomnolence. *Curr Treatment Options Neurol* 2014;16:302.

Dresler M, Spoormaker VI, Beitinger P, et al. Neuroscience-driven discovery and development of sleep therapeutics. *Pharmacol Ther* 2014;141:300–34.

Larson-Prior LJ, Ju Y, Galvin JE. Cortical–subcortical interactions in hypersomnia disorders: mechanisms underlying cognitive and behavioral aspects of the sleep–wake cycle. *Frontiers Neurol* 2014;5(165):1–13.

Morgenthaler TI, Kapur VK, Brown T, et al. Practice parameters for the treatment of narcolepsy and other hypersomnias of central origin. *Sleep* 2007;30(12):1705–11.

Stahl SM, Morrissette DA. *Stahl's illustrated sleep and wake disorders.* Cambridge: Cambridge University Press; 2016.

Disorders of Sleep and Wakefulness and their Treatment

QUESTION TWELVE

Tommy is a 32-year-old man who recently underwent diagnostic testing for obstructive sleep apnea. Results show that this patient has an apnea–hypopnea index (AHI; calculated as the total number of hypopneas and sleep apneas multiplied by 60 and divided by total sleep time (in minutes)) of 17. An AHI of 17 is indicative of:

A. No sleep apnea

B. Mild sleep apnea

C. Moderate sleep apnea

D. Severe sleep apnea

Answer to Question Twelve

The correct answer is C.

Choice	Peer answers
No sleep apnea	2%
Mild sleep apnea	20%
Moderate sleep apnea	67%
Severe sleep apnea	10%

A – Incorrect. No sleep apnea would be indicated by an AHI score of less than 5.

B – Incorrect. Mild sleep apnea is indicated by an AHI score of 5–15.

C – Correct. Moderate sleep apnea is indicated by an AHI score of 15–30.

D – Incorrect. Severe sleep apnea is indicated by an AHI score of greater than 30.

References

Epstein LJ, Kristo D, Strollo PJ, et al. Clinical guideline for the evaluation, management and long-term care of obstructive sleep apnea in adults. *J Clin Sleep Med* 2009;5(3):263–76.

Stahl SM, Morrissette DA. *Stahl's illustrated sleep and wake disorders.* Cambridge: Cambridge University Press; 2016.

QUESTION THIRTEEN

A 29-year-old male patient with shift work disorder exhibits excessive daytime sleepiness that is interfering with his ability to perform duties as an customer service agent. He is initiated on armodafinil with good therapeutic response. Modafinil, and its *R*-enantiomer armodafinil, are hypothesized to promote wakefulness and increase alertness by:

A. Decreasing norepinephrine

B. Decreasing hypocretin/orexin

C. Increasing histamine

D. All of the above

E. None of the above

Answer to Question Thirteen

The correct answer is C.

Choice	Peer answers
Decreasing norepinephrine	2%
Decreasing hypocretin/orexin	22%
Increasing histamine	45%
All of the above	13%
None of the above	18%

A – Incorrect. Modafinil and its *R*-enantiomer, armodafinil, increase both norepinephrine (NE) and dopamine (DA), possibly via their blockade of both the NE and DA reuptake transporters (NET and DAT, respectively). The actions of NE at alpha-adrenergic receptors and DA at dopamine D2 receptors are thought to contribute to the wake-promoting properties of modafinil.

B – Incorrect. Orexin/hypocretin is a key component of the arousal system; thus, the hypothesized action of modafinil and armodafinil in increasing hypocretin/orexin may help promote alertness.

C – Correct. Modafinil and its *R*-enantiomer, armodafinil, are hypothesized to indirectly increase histamine, either by reducing GABAergic inhibition of histaminergic neurons or via actions at orexinergic neurons. The increase in histamine may contribute to both the wake-promoting effects of modafinil as well as the potential of modafinil to increase alertness.

D and E – Incorrect.

References

Bogan RK. Armodafinil in the treatment of excessive sleepiness. *Expert Opin Pharmacother* 2010;11(6):993–1002.

Darwish M, Kirby M, D'Andrea DM, et al. Pharmacokinetics of armodafinil and modafinil after single and multiple doses in patients with excessive sleepiness associated with treated obstructive sleep apnea: a randomized, open-label, crossover study. *Clin Ther* 2010;32(12): 2074–87.

Erman MK, Seiden DJ, Yang R, et al. Efficacy and tolerability of armodafinil: effect on clinical condition late in the shift and overall functioning of patients with excessive sleepiness associated with shift work disorder. *JOEM* 2011;53(12):1460–5.

Morrissette DA. Twisting the night away: a review of the neurobiology, genetics, diagnosis, and treatment of shift work disorder. *CNS Spectr* 2013;18(Suppl 1):45–53.

Stahl SM, Morrissette DA. *Stahl's illustrated sleep and wake disorders*. Cambridge: Cambridge University Press; 2016.

CHAPTER PEER COMPARISON

For the Sleep/Wake Disorders section, the correct answer was selected 63% of the time.

8 ATTENTION DEFICIT HYPERACTIVITY DISORDER (ADHD) AND ITS TREATMENT

QUESTION ONE

Peter, a 35-year-old stockbroker, has been advised by his supervisor to come and see you, the company mental health consultant. His supervisor is complaining that he often comes late to appointments, is inappropriately fidgety, interrupts people during meetings, has been offensive towards coworkers, and has been known to party excessively on weeknights. Peter asserts that he is just fine; he has a lot of projects on his mind and is simply standing up for himself when speaking with others. He likes to go out in the evenings to unwind. Recognizing probable ADHD, you interview both the patient and his work buddy, who is a long-time friend. How would you start your questions?

A. Compared to his parents, how often does the patient …

B. Compared to other people his age, how often does the patient …

C. Compared to his childhood, how often does the patient …

D. Compared to his children, how often does the patient …

Answer to Question One

The correct answer is B.

Choice	Peer answers
Compared to his parents, how often does the patient …	1%
Compared to other people his age, how often does the patient …	83%
Compared to his childhood, how often does the patient …	16%
Compared to his children, how often does the patient …	0%

The symptoms of ADHD can **present differently** in patients at **different ages**. While **hyperactivity** is a main symptom in children, for example, this will frequently translate into **internal restlessness** in adults.

A and D – Incorrect. While ADHD has a strong genetic component, it is not advised to ask him first to compare himself to either his children or his parents. An accurate family history would be beneficial, however.

B – Correct. When trying to diagnose this adult patient with ADHD, it is preferable to **first** ask him to **compare his behavior** to that of **other adults his age**, as this will give a better idea of the severity of his symptoms at this time.

C – Incorrect. While it is important to obtain a medical history, the patient might not have the best recollection and might not be the best judge of his behaviors as a child.

References
Stahl SM. *Stahl's essential psychopharmacology*, fourth edition. New York, NY: Cambridge University Press; 2013. (Chapter 12)

QUESTION TWO

According to DSM-5 criteria, what is the maximum age threshold for symptom onset when making a diagnosis of attention deficit hyperactivity disorder (ADHD)?

A. 5

B. 7

C. 12

D. 15

Answer to Question Two

The correct answer is C.

Choice	Peer answers
5	3%
7	15%
12	75%
15	7%

A, B, and D – Incorrect.

C – Correct. In the fifth edition of the *Diagnostic and Statistical Manual of Mental Disorders*, the maximum age threshold for symptom onset for diagnosing ADHD changed from 7 to 12. Other revisions included the fact that, although symptoms must have been present prior to age 12, there does not have to have been impairment prior to age 12 when diagnosing someone who is older. The symptom count threshold also changed for adults (defined as age 17 and older), with 5 (instead of 6) symptoms required in the inattention and/or hyper-active/impulsive categories.

References

American Psychiatric Association. *Diagnostic and statistical manual of mental disorder*, fifth edition. Arlington, VA: American Psychiatric Publishing; 2013.

QUESTION THREE

A 15-year-old with inattentive-type attention deficit hyperactivity disorder has a hard time staying focused on the task at hand, has trouble organizing her work, and relies heavily on her mother to follow through with her homework. Problem-solving is one of the hardest tasks for her. Her difficulty with sustained attention could be related to aberrant activation in the:

A. Dorsolateral prefrontal cortex

B. Prefrontal motor cortex

C. Orbital frontal cortex

D. Supplementary motor cortex

Answer to Question Three

The correct answer is A.

Choice	Peer answers
Dorsolateral prefrontal cortex	73%
Prefrontal motor cortex	17%
Orbital frontal cortex	9%
Supplementary motor cortex	1%

A – Correct. **Sustained attention** is hypothetically modulated by the cortico-striatal–thalamic–cortical loop involving the **dorsolateral prefrontal cortex** (DLPFC). Inefficient activation of the DLPFC can lead to problems following through or finishing tasks, disorganization, and trouble sustaining mental effort; the patient exhibits all of these symptoms. The dorsal **anterior cingulate cortex** is important in regulating **selective attention**, and is associated with behaviors such as losing things, being distracted, and making careless mistakes. This area is certainly also inefficient in this patient.

B – Incorrect. The **prefrontal motor cortex** hypothetically modulates behaviors such as fidgeting, leaving one's seat, running/climbing, having trouble being quiet.

C – Incorrect. The **orbital frontal cortex** regulates impulsivity, which includes symptoms such as talking excessively, blurting things out, and interrupting others.

D – Incorrect. Finally, the **supplementary motor area** is implicated in planning motor actions; thus, this brain area would be more involved in hyperactive symptoms.

References
Arnsten AF. Fundamentals of attention-deficit/hyperactivity disorder: circuits and pathways. *J Clin Psychiatry* 2006;67 (Suppl 8):7–12.

Stahl SM. *Stahl's essential psychopharmacology*, fourth edition. New York, NY: Cambridge University Press; 2013. (Chapter 12)

Stahl SM, Mignon L. *Stahl's illustrated attention deficit hyperactivity disorder*. New York, NY: Cambridge University Press; 2009. (Chapter 1)

QUESTION FOUR

Which of the following is true regarding cortical brain development in children with ADHD compared to healthy controls?

A. The pattern (i.e., order) of cortical maturation is different

B. The timing of cortical maturation is different

C. The pattern and timing of cortical maturation are different

D. Neither the pattern nor the timing of cortical maturation are different

Answer to Question Four

The correct answer is B.

Choice	Peer answers
The pattern (i.e., order) of cortical maturation is different	8%
The timing of cortical maturation is different	36%
The pattern and timing of cortical maturation are different	50%
Neither the pattern nor the timing of cortical maturation are different	5%

Attention deficit hyperactivity disorder, or ADHD, is a neurodevelopmental disorder characterized by inattentive, hyperactive, and/or impulsive symptoms. Neuroimaging has been used to evaluate cortical maturation in children with ADHD compared to typically developing controls, specifically by comparing the age of attaining peak cortical thickness in children with and without ADHD.

A – Incorrect. Research shows that the pattern of cortical maturation is similar for children with and without ADHD. Specifically, the primary sensory and motor areas attain peak cortical thickness earlier in development than do high-order association areas such as the dorsolateral prefrontal cortex.

B – Correct. There are differences in the timing of cortical maturation between children with and without ADHD that are apparent as early as age 7. That is, cortical maturation in children with ADHD seems to lag behind that of healthy children. In fact, the median age by which 50% of the cortical points achieve peak thickness is delayed by 3 years in children with ADHD. Delay is most prominent in the superior and dorsolateral prefrontal regions, which are particularly important for control of attention and planning. Delay is also seen in subcortical structures. A large cross-sectional mega-analysis demonstrated that the delay in brain maturation is not attributable to medication use.

Interestingly, there is one brain region in which children with ADHD achieve peak cortical thickness earlier than typically developing controls: the primary motor cortex.

C and D – Incorrect.

References

Hoogman M, Bralten J, Hibar DP et al. Subcortical brain volume differences in participants with attention deficit hyperactivity disorder in children and adults: a cross-sectional mega-analysis. *Lancet Psychiatry* 2017;4(4):310–9.

Shaw P, Eckstrand K, Sharp W et al. Attention-deficit/hyperactivity disorder is characterized by a delay in cortical maturation. *Proc Natl Acad Sci* 2007;104(49):19649–54.

QUESTION FIVE

A clinician is considering treatment options for a 26–year–old man with ADHD who has a history of alcohol and marijuana abuse. Which of the following accurately explains the effects of different stimulant formulations on neuronal firing?

A. Pulsatile stimulation amplifies undesirable phasic dopamine (DA) and norepinephrine (NE) firing, which can lead to euphoria and abuse

B. Immediate-release stimulants lead to tonic firing, which can lead to euphoria and abuse

C. Tonic firing is the result of rapid receptor occupancy and fast onset of action as seen with extended-release formulations

D. Extended-release stimulants result in phasic stimulation of NE and DA signals, but this does not lead to euphoria and abuse

Answer to Question Five

The correct answer is A.

Choice	Peer answers
Pulsatile stimulation amplifies undesirable phasic dopamine (DA) and norepinephrine (NE) firing, which can lead to euphoria and abuse	43%
Immediate-release stimulants lead to tonic firing, which can lead to euphoria and abuse	22%
Tonic firing is the result of rapid receptor occupancy and fast onset of action as seen with extended-release formulations	2%
Extended-release stimulants result in phasic stimulation of NE and DA signals, but this does not lead to euphoria and abuse	32%

A – Correct. **Pulsatile** delivery of stimulants can cause a **frequent and rapid** increase in NE and DA, and this amplifies **phasic firing**. Phasic firing is hypothetically associated with **reward, feelings of euphoria**, and abuse potential.

B – Incorrect. **Immediate–release stimulants** rapidly increase DA and NE, thereby especially increasing phasic firing, not tonic firing. Therefore, immediate–release stimulants have a higher risk of abuse.

C and D – Incorrect. Extended-release formulations of stimulants lead to a **gradual and sustained** increase in NE and DA, thus enhancing **tonic firing**, which is hypothetically linked to the **therapeutic effects** of stimulants. They are amplifying tonic NE and DA signals, which are thought to be low in ADHD. The extended-release formulations **occupy the NE transporter** in the prefrontal cortex with slow enough onset and for long enough to enhance tonic NE and DA signaling; however, they do not block DA transporters fast enough or for long enough in the nucleus accumbens to increase phasic signaling, thus reducing abuse potential.

References

Stahl SM. *Stahl's essential psychopharmacology*, fourth edition. New York, NY: Cambridge University Press; 2013. (Chapter 12)

QUESTION SIX

Scarlet, a 25-year-old bartender, was diagnosed with ADHD at age 10. She has been on and off medication since then; first on immediate-release methylphenidate, then on the methylphenidate patch. She has experimented with illicit drugs during her late adolescence and is still a heavy drinker. After a few years of self-medication with alcohol and cigarettes, she is seeking medical attention again. You decide to put her on 80 mg/day of atomoxetine, one of the non-stimulant medications effective in ADHD. Why does atomoxetine lack abuse potential?

A. It decreases norepinephrine levels in the nucleus accumbens, but not in the prefrontal cortex

B. It increases dopamine levels in the prefrontal cortex, but not in the nucleus accumbens

C. It modulates serotonin levels in the raphe nucleus

D. It increases dopamine in the striatum and anterior cingulate cortex

Answer to Question Six

The correct answer is B.

Choice	Peer answers
It decreases norepinephrine levels in the nucleus accumbens, but not in the prefrontal cortex	14%
It increases dopamine levels in the prefrontal cortex, but not in the nucleus accumbens	73%
It modulates serotonin levels in the raphe nucleus	10%
It increases dopamine in the striatum and anterior cingulate cortex	3%

Atomoxetine is a selective norepinephrine reuptake inhibitor (**NET inhibitor**).

A – Incorrect. In the nucleus accumbens there are only a few NE neurons and NE transporters. **Inhibiting NET in the nucleus accumbens** will not lead to an increase in NE or DA.

B – Correct. The prefrontal cortex lacks high concentrations of DAT, so in this brain region, DA gets inactivated by NET. Therefore, **inhibiting NET in the prefrontal cortex** increases both DA and NE. As only a few NET exist in the nucleus accumbens, atomoxetine does not induce an increase in DA and NE in the nucleus accumbens, the reward center of the brain, thus atomoxetine does not have abuse potential.

C – Incorrect. Atomoxetine does not modulate serotonin levels.

D – Incorrect. The striatum and the anterior cingulate cortex are not brain areas involved in reward.

References
Stahl SM. *Stahl's essential psychopharmacology*, fourth edition. New York, NY: Cambridge University Press; 2013. (Chapter 12)

QUESTION SEVEN

A 15-year-old patient with ADHD has a rare mutation in the gene for the dopamine transporter (DAT). In deciding which treatment to initiate for this patient's ADHD, you know it will be important to avoid treatments that depend on normally functioning DAT. Which of the following drugs are transported into neurons via the dopamine transporter?

A. Amphetamine

B. Atomoxetine

C. Methylphenidate

D. A and B

E. None of the above

Answer to Question Seven

The correct answer is A.

Choice	Peer answers
Amphetamine	49%
Atomoxetine	12%
Methylphenidate	13%
A and B	14%
None of the above	12%

A – Correct. Amphetamine blocks DAT and the norepinephrine transporter (NET) by binding at the same site where the monoamines bind. Thus, amphetamine is a competitive inhibitor and pseudosubstrate for DAT and NET, such that (at least at high doses) amphetamine is actually transported into the presynaptic DA terminal.

B – Incorrect. Atomoxetine is an inhibitor of NET (binding at a site distinct from where monoamines bind), but does not have actions at DAT.

C – Incorrect. Methylphenidate blocks DAT and NET by binding at sites distinct from where monoamines bind (i.e., allosterically). Thus, it stops the transporters so that no monoamine (or methylphenidate) is transported into the neurons. This is similar to how most antidepressant reuptake inhibitors work.

D and E – Incorrect.

References

Stahl SM. *Stahl's essential psychopharmacology*, fourth edition. New York, NY: Cambridge University Press; 2013. (Chapter 12)

Stahl SM. *Stahl's essential psychopharmacology, the prescriber's guide*, sixth edition. New York, NY: Cambridge University Press; 2017.

QUESTION EIGHT

A patient with attention deficit hyperactivity disorder (ADHD) has not yet had successful treatment: he has experienced either loss of efficacy toward the end of the day or efficacy but insomnia at night. He is frustrated and wants to know what other treatment options exist. The most recently available new treatments for ADHD represent:

A. Novel neurotransmitter targets

B. New formulations of existing active ingredients

C. A and B

Answer to Question Eight

The correct answer is B.

Choice	Peer answers
Novel neurotransmitter targets	3%
New formulations of existing active ingredients	48%
A and B	48%

A – Incorrect. Investigational and recently available medications for ADHD largely still target the dopamine and/or norepinephrine system.

B – Correct. The majority of approved treatments for ADHD, and specifically new agents approved recently, are formulation variations of either amphetamine or methylphenidate: their differences lie not in the active ingredient, but rather in how that active ingredient is delivered – i.e., the release mechanism. Modified-release formulations are designed to release drug in a controlled and predictable manner that allows for a particular efficacy and safety profile. Modifying the release of drug can improve tolerability by eliminating peaks and troughs in plasma concentration, and can improve efficacy by increasing duration of action as well as by eliminating peaks and troughs.

C – Incorrect.

References
Grady MM, Stahl SM. A horse of a different color: how formulation influences medication effects. *CNS Spectr* 2012;17:63–9.

Neuroscience Education Institute. NEI Prescribe [Mobile application software]. 2017. Retrieved from http://nei.global/neiprescribeitunes.

QUESTION NINE

Rita is a 28-year-old patient with untreated ADHD. You are currently deciding between guanfacine and clonidine as potential treatments for this patient. The selective alpha 2A agonist guanfacine appears to be:

A. Less tolerated than the alpha 2 agonist clonidine

B. Better tolerated than the alpha 2 agonist clonidine

C. Less efficacious than the alpha 2 agonist clonidine

D. More efficacious than the alpha 2 agonist clonidine

Answer to Question Nine

The correct answer is B.

Choice	Peer answers
Less tolerated than the alpha 2 agonist clonidine	5%
Better tolerated than the alpha 2 agonist clonidine	78%
Less efficacious than the alpha 2 agonist clonidine	6%
More efficacious than the alpha 2 agonist clonidine	12%

There are two direct-acting agonists for alpha 2 receptors used to treat ADHD, guanfacine and clonidine. Guanfacine is relatively more selective for alpha 2A receptors than for other subtypes, whereas clonidine binds to alpha 2A, alpha 2B, and alpha 2C receptors. Clonidine also has actions on imidazoline receptors, which is thought to be responsible for some of clonidine's sedating and hypotensive actions.

A – Incorrect. Although the actions of clonidine at alpha 2A receptors exhibit therapeutic potential for ADHD, its actions at other receptors may increase side effects. By contrast, guanfacine is 15–60 times more selective for alpha 2A receptors than for α2B and α2C receptors. Additionally, guanfacine is 10 times weaker than clonidine at inducing sedation and lowering blood pressure. Thus, guanfacine is better tolerated than clonidine.

B – Correct. Guanfacine is better tolerated than clonidine.

C – Incorrect. Guanfacine is 25 times more potent in enhancing prefrontal cortical function. Thus, it can be said that guanfacine exhibits therapeutic efficacy with a reduced side-effect profile compared to clonidine.

D – Incorrect. There are no head-to-head comparisons to establish that guanfacine has superior efficacy to clonidine in ADHD.

References
Stahl SM. *Stahl's essential psychopharmacology*, fourth edition. New York, NY: Cambridge University Press; 2013. (Chapter 12)

Stahl SM. *Stahl's essential psychopharmacology, the prescriber's guide*, sixth edition. New York, NY: Cambridge University Press; 2017.

QUESTION TEN

Aggregate data suggest that, compared to stimulants, non–stimulants have:

A. Smaller effect sizes

B. Approximately the same effect sizes

C. Larger effect sizes

Answer to Question Ten

The correct answer is A.

Choice	Peer answers
Smaller effect sizes	90%
Approximately the same effect sizes	17%
Larger effect sizes	3%

A – Correct. Multiple meta-analyses assessing the effects of stimulant medications have shown that, as a class, non-stimulants have smaller effect sizes than stimulants. Due to differences in study design, these meta-analyses do not address potential differences in efficacy among specific medications.

B and C – Incorrect.

References
Faraone SV, Glatt SJ. A comparison of the efficacy of medications for adult attention-deficit/hyperactivity disorder using meta-analysis of effect sizes. *J Clin Psychiatry* 2010;71(6):754–63.

Faraone SV, Biederman J, Spencer TJ, Aleardi M. Comparing the efficacy of medications for ADHD using meta-analysis. *MedGenMed* 2006;8(4):4.

Hanwella R, Senanayake M, de Silva V. Comparative efficacy and acceptability of methylphenidate and atomoxetine in treatment of attention deficit hyperactivity disorder in children and adolescents: a meta-analysis. *BMC Psychiatry* 2011;11:176.

QUESTION ELEVEN

A 44-year-old man was diagnosed with ADHD-inattentive subtype in college but has not taken medication for the last several years. He is seeking treatment now because of declining work performance following a promotion 7 months ago. Specifically, he complains of difficulty finishing a paper and staying focused during meetings and fears that his boss is losing confidence in him. Assessment confirms a diagnosis of ADHD-inattentive subtype. After 2 months treatment on a therapeutic dose of a long-acting stimulant, he states that his focus, sustained attention, and distractibility are much better, but that he still can't get organized and that it takes him longer to complete tasks than it should. At this point, would it be appropriate to raise the dose of the stimulant to try to address his residual symptoms?

A. Yes

B. No

Answer to Question Eleven

The correct answer is B.

Choice	Peer answers
Yes	58%
No	42%

A – Incorrect. Dose–response studies of stimulant medications suggest that the optimal dose varies across individuals and depends somewhat on the domain of function. Specifically, higher doses may lead to greater improvement of some domains (e.g., vigilance, attention) but not executive function (e.g., planning, cognitive flexibility, inhibitory control).

B – Correct. If medication dose is high enough to substantially diminish symptoms of inattention and distractibility, then executive function needs to be addressed independently and will not likely respond to higher medication dosing.

References

Pietrzak RH, Mollica CM, Maruff P, Snyder PJ. Cognitive effects of immediate-release methylphenidate in children with attention-deficit/hyperactivity disorder. *Neurosci Biobehav Rev* 2006;30:1225–45.

Swanson J, Baler MD, Volkow ND. Understanding the effects of stimulant medications on cognition individuals with attention-deficit hyperactivity disorder: a decade of progress. *Neuropsychopharmacology* 2011;36:207–26.

QUESTION TWELVE

The cumulative data on the effects of physical exercise as an adjunctive treatment for children with ADHD have demonstrated the potential beneficial effects of:

A. Acute aerobic exercise

B. Chronic aerobic exercise

C. A and B

D. Neither A nor B

Answer to Question Twelve

The correct answer is C.

Choice	Peer answers
Acute aerobic exercise	13%
Chronic aerobic exercise	22%
A and B	59%
Neither A nor B	6%

A and B – Partially correct.

C – Correct. Comparisons have been made between aerobic/nonaerobic, and acute vs. chronic exercise on cognitive and behavioral symptoms in children with ADHD. Numerous published studies on exercise and cognition in children with ADHD have shown that aerobic exercise appears to be the most effective for improvements in executive function (EF). Both acute and chronic exercise have beneficial effects on behavioral and cognitive measures in children with ADHD, when assessed immediately after exercise. Cognitive measures include improved response inhibition, cognitive control, attention allocation, cognitive flexibility, processing speed, and vigilance.

Physical exercise is beneficial as adjunctive treatment, but there's not enough evidence to suggest that it is a stand-alone treatment. Exercise may be particularly effective for youth, potentially preventing or altering the course of ADHD. The literature is promising; however, the most challenging complications for these types of studies are: random assignment, blinded raters, and adequate control groups.

D – Incorrect.

References

Den Heijer AE, **Groen Y**, **Tucha L** et al. Sweat it out? The effects of physical exercise on cognition and behavior in children and adults with ADHD: a systematic literature review. *J Neural Transm (Vienna)* 2017;124(Suppl 1):3–26.

Hoza B, **Martin CP**, **Pirog A**, et al. Using physical activity to manage ADHD symptoms: The state of the evidence. *Curr Psychiatry Rep* 2016;18(12):113.

QUESTION THIRTEEN

A patient with a history of alcohol use disorder has been sober for 6 weeks. He begins medication treatment for adult attention deficit hyperactivity disorder (ADHD) and experiences improvement, but 4 months later relapses with his alcohol use disorder, engaging in three binge-drinking episodes over a 2-week period. Does this patient need to discontinue medication treatment for ADHD?

A. Yes, he should be switched to non-medication treatment

B. Only if he is currently on a long-acting stimulant; non-stimulant medication is acceptable in this scenario

C. No, both long-acting stimulants and non–stimulant medications are acceptable in this scenario

Answer to Question Thirteen

The correct answer is C.

Choice	Peer answers
Yes, he should be switched to non-medication treatment	12%
Only if he is currently on a long-acting stimulant; non-stimulant medication is acceptable in this scenario	27%
No, both long-acting stimulants and non-stimulant medications are acceptable in this scenario	62%

Because ongoing substance abuse can hinder the treatment progress of other disorders, in many cases it may be necessary to address this problem first. However, although these are general guidelines in the ordering of treatment, one should be careful that this prioritization of symptoms/conditions does not lead to the neglect of ADHD treatment in adults.

A – Incorrect. Atomoxetine, which is approved for adult ADHD, has been shown to be effective for ADHD and to decrease both alcohol cravings and heavy drinking days. Atomoxetine is not contraindicated in patients with acute alcohol use disorder or in patients with liver impairment, so the patient's alcohol use would not require medication discontinuation. Thus, it is an appropriate treatment choice; however, it is not the only appropriate treatment choice.

B – Incorrect. Long-acting stimulant medications are not contraindicated in patients with acute alcohol use disorder, although they do carry a black-box warning indicating caution in patients with history of substance dependence. In general, non-stimulant options may be preferable to stimulants in patients with substance use disorders, but long-acting stimulants should remain as a second-tier option.

C – Correct. Non-stimulant and long-acting stimulant medications are both options for ADHD co-occurring with substance use disorders; however, non-stimulants may be preferred as the first-line approach. If a stimulant is prescribed to a patient in early sobriety from substance use and/or continued low-level substance use, then he/she should be monitored closely for misuse of the prescribed medication.

References

McGough JJ. Treatment controversies in adult ADHD. *Am J Psychiatry* 2016;173:960–6.

Wilens TE, Morrison NR. The intersection of attention-deficit/hyperactivity disorder and substance abuse. *Curr Opin Psychiatry* 2011;24:280–5.

Wilens TE, Morrison NR, Prince J. An update on the pharmacotherapy of attention-deficit/hyperactivity disorder in adults. *Expert Rev Neurother* 2011;11(10):1443–65.

QUESTION FOURTEEN

A 7-year-old boy has just been diagnosed with attention deficit hyperactivity disorder (ADHD), combined type, and his care provider feels that the best therapeutic choice is a stimulant. Family history is significant for depression and diabetes. The patient's medical history is significant for asthma; physical exam reveals no abnormalities. According to current recommendations, what should be the care provider's next step?

A. Prescribe a stimulant, as no additional tests are indicated for this patient

B. Obtain an electrocardiogram (ECG), as this patient's family history and exam results warrant it

C. Obtain an ECG, as this is mandatory prior to prescribing a stimulant to any child

D. Prescribe a non-stimulant, as a stimulant would not be appropriate for this patient

Answer to Question Fourteen

The correct answer is A.

Choice	Peer answers
Prescribe a stimulant, as no additional tests are indicated for this patient	72%
Obtain an electrocardiogram (ECG), as this patient's family history and exam results warrant it	6%
Obtain an ECG, as this is mandatory prior to prescribing a stimulant to any child	16%
Prescribe a non-stimulant, as a stimulant would not be appropriate for this patient	5%

A – Correct. Current recommendations from the American Heart Association (AHA) are that it is reasonable but not mandatory to obtain an electrocardiogram (ECG) prior to prescribing a stimulant to a child. The American Academy of Pediatrics (AAP) does not recommend an ECG prior to starting a stimulant for most children.

B – Incorrect. According to recommendations, it is at the physician's discretion whether or not to obtain an ECG; however, in this case there is no evidence of cardiovascular disease in either the family history or patient exam.

C – Incorrect. According to AHA and AAP recommendations, treatment with a stimulant should not be withheld because an ECG is not obtained.

D – Incorrect. There is no reason why a stimulant would not be a reasonable choice for this patient.

References

American Academy of Pediatrics/American Heart Association. American Academy of Pediatrics/American Heart Association clarification of statement on cardiovascular evaluation and monitoring of children and adolescents with heart disease receiving medications for ADHD. *J Dev Behav Pediatr* 2008;29(4):335.

CHAPTER PEER COMPARISON

For the ADHD section, the correct answer was selected 62% of the time.

9 DEMENTIA AND COGNITIVE FUNCTION AND ITS TREATMENT

QUESTION ONE

Mary, a 79-year-old patient, is brought to your office by her daughter, who reports that her mother has been exhibiting several concerning symptoms over the past year. Comprehensive questioning reveals that her symptoms are: trouble remembering familiar things, such as telephone numbers commonly dialed; not recognizing some close family members who visit often; and difficulty performing writing tasks. The patient's motor function appears to be unaffected. Although not definitive, these symptoms are most likely indicative of which type of dementia?

A. Alzheimer's disease

B. Dementia with Lewy bodies

C. Huntington's disease

D. Frontotemporal dementia

Answer to Question One

The correct answer is A.

Choice	Peer answers
Alzheimer's disease	94%
Dementia with Lewy bodies	2%
Huntington's disease	0%
Frontotemporal dementia	4%

Differential diagnosis of dementias can be difficult, as all are characterized by the core symptom of memory impairment. However, it may be possible to distinguish dementias clinically through other presenting symptoms.

A – Correct. In addition to memory impairment, Alzheimer's disease consists of deficits in language (aphasia), motor function (apraxia), recognition (agnosia), or executive functioning, all of which this patient exhibits. Definitive diagnosis, however, is not possible until autopsy.

B – Incorrect. Dementia with Lewy bodies is often accompanied by extrapyramidal symptoms, which this patient does not have.

C – Incorrect. Huntington's disease is associated with spasmodic movements and incoordination, which are also absent in this patient.

D – Incorrect. In frontotemporal dementia, patients often are disinhibited and may be extremely talkative, symptoms that are also not part of this patient's presentation.

References

Stahl SM. *Stahl's essential psychopharmacology*, fourth edition. New York, NY: Cambridge University Press; 2013. (Chapter 13)

QUESTION TWO

A young man who is pre-med and has a family history of Alzheimer's disease is interested in learning more about the brain regions involved in memory and the development of Alzheimer's disease. You describe the pathways of acetylcholine, an important neurotransmitter involved in dementia. As part of your explanation, you tell him that major cholinergic projections stem from the _____ to the _____, which are believed to be involved in memory.

A. Basal forebrain; nucleus accumbens

B. Basal forebrain; hippocampus

C. Striatum; hypothalamus

D. Striatum; prefrontal cortex

Answer to Question Two

The correct answer is B.

Choice	Peer answers
Basal forebrain; nucleus accumbens	10%
Basal forebrain; hippocampus	70%
Striatum; hypothalamus	6%
Striatum; prefrontal cortex	14%

A, C, and D – Incorrect.

B – Correct. Acetylcholine is an important neurotransmitter, and is thought to be involved in memory. Major acetylcholine neurotransmitter projections originating in the basal forebrain project to the prefrontal cortex, amygdala, and hippocampus, the primary brain structure involved in short-term memory and most greatly affected in Alzheimer's disease.

References

Stahl SM. *Stahl's essential psychopharmacology*, fourth edition. New York, NY: Cambridge University Press; 2013. (Chapter 13)

Woolf NJ, **Butcher LL**. Cholinergic systems mediate action from movement to higher consciousness. *Behav Brain Res* 2011;221(2): 488–98.

QUESTION THREE

A young woman brings her 72-year-old mother for an appointment because she is concerned that her mother may have Alzheimer's disease. The mother does not feel that anything is wrong, but her daughter states that she has seemed somewhat depressed and forgetful lately. Data have shown that:

A. Depression is often comorbid with Alzheimer's disease

B. Depression may increase the risk of developing Alzheimer's disease

C. Depression may be a prodromal symptom of Alzheimer's disease

D. All of the above

E. None of the above

Answer to Question Three

The correct answer is D.

Choice	Peer answers
Depression is often comorbid with Alzheimer's disease	5%
Depression may increase the risk of developing Alzheimer's disease	0%
Depression may be a prodromal symptom of Alzheimer's disease	7%
All of the above	86%
None of the above	2%

A – Partially correct. Mood symptoms can occur as part of Alzheimer's disease and in fact are typically the first notable symptom (often manifested as apathy rather than sadness). In addition, depression is a common comorbid illness in patients with Alzheimer's disease.

B – Partially correct. Depression has been hypothesized to be a possible risk factor for Alzheimer's disease.

C – Partially correct. Depression has been hypothesized to be a possible prodromal symptom of Alzheimer's disease, with some evidence suggesting that it may exacerbate the progression of Alzheimer's pathology.

D – Correct (all of the above).

E – Incorrect (none of the above).

References

Barnes DE, Yaffe K, Byers AL, et al. Midlife vs late-life depressive symptoms and risk of dementia: differential effects for Alzheimer disease and vascular dementia. *Arch Gen Psychiatry* 2012;69(5):493–8.

Pomara N, Bruno D, Sarreal AS, et al. Lower CSF amyloid beta peptides and higher F2-isoprostanes in cognitively intact elderly individuals with major depressive disorder. *Am J Psychiatry* 2012;169: 523–30.

QUESTION FOUR

Thomas is a 54-year-old man with a family history of Alzheimer's disease. As a voluntary participant in research studies on Alzheimer's disease, Thomas recently had amyloid positron emission tomography (amyloid PET) neuroimaging done. Although he currently exhibits no behavioral symptoms of Alzheimer's disease, Thomas's amyloid PET scans revealed accumulation of beta amyloid protein throughout cortical and limbic areas of his brain. Although much research is yet to be done, data indicate that the normal physiological role of amyloid beta protein may include:

A. Blood vessel repair functions

B. Antimicrobial functions

C. Both of the above

Answer to Question Four

The correct answer is C.

Choice	Peer answers
Blood vessel repair functions	28%
Antimicrobial functions	4%
Both of the above	68%

A – Partially correct. One hypothesis posits that amyloid beta may act as a sealant at sites of injury or leakage on vessel walls. In this way, amyloid beta may protect from acute brain injury; however, the accumulation of amyloid is associated with development of dementia.

B – Partially correct. Evidence indicates that amyloid beta may have antimicrobial functions. During microbial infection, adhesion of microbes to the host cell is mediated by carbohydrates found in the microbial cell wall. Amyloid beta oligomers bind to cell wall microbial carbohydrates, preventing microbes from adhering to the host cell. This binding of amyloid beta to the microbial cell wall also induces fibrillization of amyloid beta, encompassing microbes and causing agglutination (clumping of microbes so that they can be more readily removed by phagocytosis).

C – Correct. Both blood vessel repair and antimicrobial actions are hypothesized to be normal physiological roles for amyloid beta protein.

References

Atwood CS, Bishop GM, Perry G et al. Amyloid beta: a vascular sealant that protects against hemorrhage? *J Neurosci Res* 2002;70(3):356.

Kokjohn TA, Maarfouf CL, Roher AE. Is Alzheimer's disease amyloidosis the result of a repair mechanism gone astray? *Alzheimer's Dementia* 2012;8(6):574–83.

Kumar DK, Choi SH, Washicosky KJ et al. Amyloid–beta peptide protects against microbial infection in mouse and worm models of Alzheimer's disease. *Sci Transl Med* 2016;8(340):340ra72.

QUESTION FIVE

A 68-year-old patient with an early diagnosis of Alzheimer's disease is put on a cholinesterase inhibitor in hopes of improving his cognitive function. This patient has been a chain smoker for over 40 years and refuses to give up the habit. Which of the following medications would *not* be appropriate for this patient, given his smoking habit?

A. Donepezil

B. Galantamine

C. Rivastigmine

D. None of these medications should be prescribed to a patient who smokes

E. There are no contraindications due to smoking for these medications

Answer to Question Five

The correct answer is E.

Choice	Peer answers
Donepezil	8%
Galantamine	9%
Rivastigmine	11%
None of these medications should be prescribed to a patient who smokes	4%
There are no contraindications due to smoking for these medications	68%

A – Incorrect. Donepezil, a reversible, long-acting selective inhibitor of acetylcholinesterase (AChE), may be a good choice, resulting in mainly transient gastrointestinal side effects.

B – Incorrect. Galantamine has a dual mechanism of action: AChE inhibition and positive allosteric modulation (PAM) of nicotinic cholinergic receptors. This may be a good choice for this patient.

C – Incorrect. Rivastigmine, delivered both orally and via a transdermal formulation, has similar safety and efficacy as donepezil. The oral formulation may result in more gastrointestinal side effects than donepezil, owing to its pharmacokinetic profile and inhibition of both AChE and butyrylcholinesterase (BuChE) in the periphery.

D – Incorrect.

E – Correct. One can potentially choose any cholinesterase inhibitor as a first-line treatment, because specific contraindications due to smoking do not presently appear in the literature.

References
Stahl SM. *Stahl's essential psychopharmacology*, fourth edition. New York, NY: Cambridge University Press; 2013. (Chapter 13)

Stahl SM. *Stahl's essential psychopharmacology, the prescriber's guide*, fifth edition. New York, NY: Cambridge University Press; 2014.

QUESTION SIX

John, a 73-year-old mid-stage Alzheimer's patient, has been on done-pezil, 10 mg/day for approximately 8 months to aid in improving his cognitive functioning. His wife has begun to notice a loss of effectiveness over the past month, and they present today to determine a new course of action. You decide to augment John's donepezil with 5 mg/day of memantine. Which of the following properties of memantine may be useful in treating Alzheimer's disease?

A. Serotonin 3 (5HT3) antagonism

B. Sigma antagonism

C. *N*-methyl-D-aspartate (NMDA) antagonism

D. NMDA antagonism at the magnesium site

Answer to Question Six

The correct answer is D.

Choice	Peer answers
Serotonin 3 (5HT3) antagonism	4%
Sigma antagonism	1%
N-methyl-D-aspartate (NMDA) antagonism	55%
NMDA antagonism at the magnesium site	39%

A and B – Incorrect. Memantine possesses weak 5HT3 antagonist properties and sigma antagonist properties, but it is currently unclear if these contribute to its benefit in Alzheimer's disease.

C – Incorrect. Memantine is an NMDA antagonist, but it does not bind at the PCP site.

D – Correct. Memantine is an NMDA antagonist that binds to the magnesium site. It works as an uncompetitive open-channel NDMA receptor antagonist (i.e., low–moderate affinity, voltage dependence, fast-blocking/unblocking kinetics). Memantine is quickly reversible if phasic bursts of glutamate occurs, but is able to block tonic glutamate release from having negative downstream effects. This hypothetically stops the excessive glutamate from interfering with the resting glutamate neuron's physiological activity and thus improving memory.

References

Kotermanski SE, Johnson JW. Mg2+ imparts NMDA receptor subtype selectivity to the Alzheimer's drug memantine. *J Neurosci* 2009;29(9): 2774–9.

Stahl SM. *Stahl's essential psychopharmacology*, fourth edition. New York, NY: Cambridge University Press; 2013. (Chapter 13)

QUESTION SEVEN

Mildred is a 66-year-old patient. She is currently showing no signs of Alzheimer's disease but is considering enrolling in one of the ongoing Alzheimer's disease immunotherapy-based clinical trials (the DIAN-TU and A4 studies). You explain to Mildred that such immunotherapy involves:

A. Antibodies that bind to NMDA receptors in the brain

B. Antibodies that bind to amyloid protein in the brain

C. Antibodies that bind to hyperphosphorylated tau in the blood

Answer to Question Seven

The correct answer is B.

Choice	Peer answers
Antibodies that bind to NMDA receptors in the brain	6%
Antibodies that bind to amyloid protein in the brain	69%
Antibodies that bind to hyperphosphorylated tau in the blood	25%

One of the main hypotheses regarding the neuropathology of Alzheimer's disease is the "amyloid cascade hypothesis." The amyloid cascade hypothesis proposes that the overproduction, or impaired clearance, of a protein called amyloid beta leads to a cascade of events including aggregation of amyloid beta into plaques, hyperphosphorylation of tau protein, formation of neurofibrillary tangles, synaptic failure, neuron loss, and eventually, memory deficits and severe cognitive dysfunction. Most pharmacological agents that have been developed and tested over the recent past are based on this amyloid cascade hypothesis. There are several clinical trials underway that are taking advantage of our emerging ability to predict, and possibly prevent, the development of Alzheimer's disease at the preclinical stage, prior to even mild cognitive impairment by preventing the accumulation of amyloid beta. These include the Dominantly Inherited Alzheimer Network Trials Unit (DIAN-TU) and the Anti-Amyloid Treatment in Asymptomatic Alzheimer's (A4) study.

A – Incorrect. Although the currently available Alzheimer's drug memantine acts by antagonizing NMDA receptors, the ongoing DIAN-TU and A4 clinical trials do not involve antibodies that bind to NMDA receptors.

B – Correct. The ongoing immunotherapy clinical trials (DIAN-TU and A4) utilize various antibodies that bind to different portions or conformations of the amyloid beta peptide and are thought to remove amyloid beta from the brain via three hypothesized mechanisms. These mechanisms include: peripheral sink; disaggregation; and microglia engagement and phagocytosis.

C – Incorrect. There are some Alzheimer's disease experts who do not support the idea that amyloid beta is the driving protein behind amyloid pathology. Many such researchers hypothesize that an effective treatment strategy for Alzheimer's disease will need to include therapeutic agents that target and remove tau protein. This hypothesis is being actively pursued in the development of antibodies that bind to tau proteins in the cerebrospinal fluid. However, the ongoing immunotherapy clinical trials (DIAN-TU and A4) do not currently involve antibodies that bind to tau protein in the cerebrospinal fluid or the blood.

References

Alzheimer's Association. 2016 Alzheimer's disease facts and figures. *Alzheimer's Dement* 2016;12(4):459–509.

Godyń J, Jończyk J, Panek D et al. Therapeutic strategies for Alzheimer's disease in clinical trials. *Pharmacol Res* 2016;68:127–38.

Harrison JR, Owen MJ. Alzheimer's disease: the amyloid hypothesis on trial. *Br J Psychiatry* 2016;208(1):1–3.

Panza F, Seripa D, Solfrizzi V et al. Emerging drugs to reduce abnormal β-amyloid protein in Alzheimer's disease patients. *Expert Opin Emerg Drugs* 2016;21(4): 377–91.

For more information about ongoing Alzheimer's disease clinical trials, including how to enroll in the A4, DIAN-TU, and other studies, please visit the following resources:

www.nia.nih.gov/alzheimers/clinical-trials

https://dian.wustl.edu/our-research/observational-study/

Dementia and Cognitive Function and its Treatment

QUESTION EIGHT

Sam, a 49-year-old patient, is in your office today for a consultation. He admits that he has had a significant lack of interest in golfing, one of his favorite past-times; he is frustrated that it has become seemingly more difficult to swing the club. In addition, he notes that he has recently become increasingly agitated when other church parishioners sit in the seat that he prefers during the church service and has even verbally lashed out at them. With this information, how might you best describe Sam's symptoms?

A. Early stages of Alzheimer's disease, focusing on mood changes

B. Depression–executive dysfunction

C. Amnestic mild cognitive impairment

D. Natural aging/elderly disposition symptoms

Answer to Question Eight

The correct answer is B.

Choice	Peer answers
Early stages of Alzheimer's disease, focusing on mood changes	26%
Depression–executive dysfunction	68%
Amnestic mild cognitive impairment	1%
Natural aging/elderly disposition symptoms	5%

A – Incorrect. Early stages of Alzheimer's may be difficult to diagnose and distinguish from depression–executive dysfunction at this point, but cognitive impairment is not quite apparent. In addition, he is well aware of his own symptoms, which is frequently not the case with Alzheimer's disease.

B – Correct. Late-onset depression may be a dysfunction of prefrontal cortico-striatal–thalamic–cortical (CSTC) circuits in relation to executive dysfunction. This may be termed depression–executive dysfunction, or DED, and is characterized by psychomotor retardation, reduced interested in activities, impaired insight, and pronounced behavioral disability. Often times an episode of depression may be confused with dementia in the elderly.

C – Incorrect. Amnestic mild cognitive impairment (MCI) is defined as a memory impairment compared to age-matched peers with normal cognitive function in other domains (no aphasia, apraxia, agnosia, or executive dysfunction) and no functional evidence of actual dementia. As this patient is having problems with apraxia and agitation, this is likely not the correct diagnosis.

D – Incorrect. Natural aging would likely not include agitation and aggression, as described here.

References

Alexopoulos GS, Kiosses DN, Heo M, Murphy CF, Shanmugham B, Gunning-Dixon F. Executive dysfunction and the course of geriatric depression. *Biol Psychiatry* 2005;58(3):204–10.

Stahl SM. *Stahl's essential psychopharmacology*, fourth edition. New York, NY: Cambridge University Press; 2013.(Chapter 13)

QUESTION NINE

A 79-year-old man presents to your office with his wife. She lists significant medical history, such as chronic renal failure, mild cirrhosis, arrhythmia, and a recent diagnosis of moderately severe Alzheimer's disease by their family physician. Which of the following medications for Alzheimer's disease has a "do not use" warning for patients with renal and hepatic impairment?

A. Donepezil

B. Rivastigmine

C. Memantine

D. Galantamine

Answer to Question Nine

The correct answer is D.

Choice	Peer answers
Donepezil	14%
Rivastigmine	22%
Memantine	15%
Galantamine	49%

A – Incorrect. Donepezil, a cholinesterase inhibitor, could potentially be given to this patient to aid in treatment of Alzheimer's, although little data has been gathered on its effects in regard to renal and hepatic impairment. Cardiac patients should use this drug with caution due to reports of syncopal episodes.

B – Incorrect. Rivastigmine, a cholinesterase inhibitor, appears as though it could be useful in this situation, as it can be used in patients with renal or hepatic impairment; caution should be exercised in cardiac patients due to potential syncopal episodes.

C – Incorrect. Memantine, an NMDA receptor antagonist, would be useful in this case due to its indication of approval for treatment of moderate to severe dementia, with which this patient has been diagnosed, although the label indicates a lowered dose for use in severe renal impairment. However, there is not likely to be a problem for hepatic- or cardiac-impaired patients.

D – Correct. Galantamine has a "do not use" warning in patients with renal and hepatic impairment, as well as a caution warning when used in cardiac-impaired patients. Furthermore, galantamine, a cholinesterase inhibitor, is often prescribed as one of the first-line treatments for early stage Alzheimer's, rather than moderately severe cases.

References

Stahl SM. *Stahl's essential psychopharmacology*, fourth edition. New York, NY: Cambridge University Press; 2013. (Chapter 13)

QUESTION TEN

Virgil is a 65-year-old man. His daughter reports that he began for-getting birthdays, grandchildren's names, and other important infor-mation approximately 1 year ago and that he has become increasingly unable to perform many activities, such as paying bills on time. Neuropsychiatric testing shows moderate cognitive impairment not attributable to any medical or psychiatric condition. Virgil has never been tested for biomarkers of Alzheimer's disease, but genetic testing has revealed that he carries an Alzheimer's-associated mutation in the presenilin gene. What would be the most likely diagnosis for this patient according to the National Institute on Aging and Alzheimer's Association 2011 diagnostic criteria for dementia?

A. Possible Alzheimer's dementia

B. Probable Alzheimer's dementia with increased level of certainty

C. Alzheimer's dementia

Answer to Question Ten

The correct answer is B.

Choice	Peer answers
Possible Alzheimer's dementia	10%
Probable Alzheimer's dementia with increased level of certainty	77%
Alzheimer's dementia	13%

A – Incorrect. The diagnosis of "possible Alzheimer's dementia" is reserved for individuals who exhibit dementia with an atypical course and mixed presentation, which is not demonstrated in this patient's case. In instances where the dementia is atypical or mixed in its presentation, and especially without biomarker evidence, such dementia could be due to Alzheimer's disease, Lewy body dementia, vascular dementia, or frontotemporal dementia (or some combination of the pathologies associated with each of these dementia types).

B – Correct. This patient is exhibiting the typical symptoms of Alzheimer's dementia including an insidious onset, with a history of worsening cognition, amnesic symptoms, and deficits in executive function being the most prominent symptoms. Although biomarker evidence (including positive amyloid PET neuroimaging and increased cerebrospinal fluid tau levels) would increase the certainty of the diagnosis, the fact that this patient carries the Alzheimer's disease-associated presenilin mutation allows us to make the diagnosis of "probable Alzheimer's dementia with increased level of certainty."

C – Incorrect. The only way to currently make a confirmed diagnosis of Alzheimer's dementia is through post-mortem visualization of Alzheimer's neuropathology.

References

McKhann GM, Knopman DS, Chertkow H et al. The diagnosis of dementia due to Alzheimer's disease: recommendations from the National Institute on Aging–Alzheimer's Association workgroups on diagnostic guidelines for Alzheimer's disease. *Alzheimers Dement* 2011;7(3):263–9.

QUESTION ELEVEN

A 65-year-old woman is concerned that her husband is exhibiting some symptoms suggestive of Alzheimer's disease. She is extremely anxious and wants a definitive diagnosis. Which of the following is true regarding the current application of biomarkers for the early detection and differential diagnosis of Alzheimer's disease?

A. There are currently no biomarkers that can identify Alzheimer's pathology

B. Use of biomarkers in Alzheimer's disease is currently recommended solely for research purposes

C. Biomarkers are now being used to diagnose Alzheimer's disease in clinical practice

Answer to Question Eleven

The correct answer is B.

Choice	Peer answers
There are currently no biomarkers that can identify Alzheimer's pathology	9%
Use of biomarkers in Alzheimer's disease is currently recommended solely for research purposes	74%
Biomarkers are now being used to diagnose Alzheimer's disease in clinical practice	17%

One difficulty in the diagnosis and early treatment of Alzheimer's disease is that diagnostic criteria require both clinical evidence and post-mortem identification of plaques and tangles. As the clinical manifestation of Alzheimer's disease likely occurs years after the initial deposition of beta amyloid, when disease course is probably still modifiable, *in vivo* detection of Alzheimer pathology is critical for the early detection and management of Alzheimer's disease. Over the past decade, there have been numerous developments in the detection of Alzheimer pathology *in vivo*. Biomarkers for Alzheimer's disease include cerebrospinal fluid (CSF) measures of beta amyloid and tau, magnetic resonance imaging (MRI) of brain atrophy, and visualization of beta amyloid and glucose metabolism using special tracers coupled with positron emission tomography (PET). Use of these biomarkers has been shown to predict those who are likely to progress from asymptomatic phases and mild cognitive impairment to full-blown dementia.

A and C – Incorrect.

B – Correct. The National Institute on Aging–Alzheimer's Association workgroup recently published revised diagnostic guidelines that utilize these biomarkers for the early detection of Alzheimer pathology and differential diagnosis of Alzheimer's disease. Although the use of biomarkers for Alzheimer's disease is currently recommended solely for research and clinical trial applications, there is great hope that these biomarkers will become clinically relevant in the near future.

References

Cummings JL. Biomarkers in Alzheimer's disease drug development. *Alzheimer Dementia* 2011;7:e13–44.

McKhann GM, Knopman DS, Chertkow H, et al. The diagnosis of dementia due to Alzheimer's disease: recommendations from the National Institute on Aging–Alzheimer's Association workgroups on diagnostic guidelines for Alzheimer's disease. *Alzheimer Dementia* 2011;7: 263–9.

Sperling RA, **Aisen PS**, **Beckett LA**, et al. Toward defining the preclinical stages of Alzheimer's disease: recommendations from the National Institute on Aging–Alzheimer's Association workgroups on diagnostic guidelines for Alzheimer's disease. *Alzheimer Dementia* 2011;7: 280–92.

Dementia and Cognitive Function and its Treatment

QUESTION TWELVE

An 87-year-old patient with mild cognitive impairment is suspected of being in the early, prodromal stage of Alzheimer's disease. Although currently for research purposes, which biomarker evidence would support a diagnosis of Alzheimer's disease?

A. Decreased cerebrospinal fluid (CSF) levels of amyloid beta and increased CSF levels of tau protein

B. Decreased levels of brain amyloid beta on positron emission tomography (PET) scans

C. Both of the above

D. Neither of the above

Answer to Question Twelve

The correct answer is A.

Choice	Peer answers
Decreased cerebrospinal fluid (CSF) levels of amyloid beta and increased CSF levels of tau protein	55%
Decreased levels of brain amyloid beta on positron emission tomography (PET) scans	3%
Both of the above	19%
Neither of the above	23%

A – Correct. During the presymptomatic stage of Alzheimer's disease, A-beta peptides are slowly and relentlessly deposited into the brain rather than eliminated via the CSF, plasma, and liver. As Alzheimer's disease progresses, tau and phosphorylated tau protein levels in the CSF increase. Low CSF levels of A-beta and high levels of CSF tau can therefore be used as a biomarkers of Alzheimer's disease.

B – Incorrect. Levels of brain amyloid beta can be detected with PET scans using radioactive neuroimaging tracers that bind to the fibrillar form of amyloid and thus label mature neuritic plaques. In normal controls, amyloid PET imaging shows the absence of amyloid. However, individuals who are cognitively normal may have moderate accumulation of amyloid; these individuals are likely in the presymptomatic first stage of Alzheimer's disease. In the final stage of Alzheimer's disease, when full-blown dementia is clinically evident, a large accumulation of brain amyloid can readily be seen.

References

Stahl SM. *Stahl's essential psychopharmacology*, fourth edition. New York, NY: Cambridge University Press; 2013. (Chapter 13)

QUESTION THIRTEEN

William is a 77-year-old patient with mid- to late-stage Alzheimer's disease. His behavioral impairment has drastically worsened over the past month. The patient's family is concerned that William's rapidly deteriorating psychiatric and physical functioning may be due to his medication (donepezil 10 mg/day) no longer working. The treating clinician feels that Alzheimer's disease may not be the primary cause of William's recent deterioration. Which comorbid illness most commonly goes undetected in patients with moderate to severe dementia?

A. Bacteriuria

B. Dehydration

C. Hypothyroidism

Answer to Question Thirteen

The correct answer is A.

Choice	Peer answers
Bacteriuria	69%
Dehydration	20%
Hypothyroidism	11%

A – Correct. Nearly 40% of individuals with dementia may be suffering from an undetected but modifiable illness. Bacteriuria is the most common undiagnosed illness in patients suffering from dementia, and it can lead to incontinence and increased agitation.

B – Incorrect. Although untreated dehydration has been found in 3% of individuals with dementia, it is not the most common undetected comorbid illness.

C – Incorrect. Although untreated hypothyroidism has been found in 1–3% of individuals with dementia, it is not the most common undetected comorbid illness.

References

Hodgson NA, Gitlin LN, Winter L, et al. Undiagnosed illness and neuropsychiatric behaviors in community residing older adults with dementia. *Alzheimer Dis Assoc Disord* 2011;25:109–15.

CHAPTER PEER COMPARISON

For the Dementia and Cognitive Function section, the correct answer was selected 68% of the time.

10 SUBSTANCE USE AND IMPULSIVE COMPULSIVE DISORDERS AND THEIR TREATMENT

QUESTION ONE

Your 16-year-old son is thrilled when he wins the 100-meter dash in an important high school competition. This "natural high" is most likely associated with inducing dopamine release in his mesolimbic pathway and in his:

A. Hypothalamus

B. Amygdala

C. Hippocampus

D. Cerebellum

E. Motor cortex

Answer to Question One

The correct answer is B.

Choice	Peer answers
Hypothalamus	15%
Amygdala	64%
Hippocampus	15%
Cerebellum	2%
Motor cortex	4%

A, C, D, and E – Incorrect. These brain regions are not known to be directly involved in the reactive reward system.

B – Correct. The brain can experience a "natural high" from activities such as athletic or intellectual accomplishments. This occurs when dopamine neurons release dopamine in the mesolimbic pathway, which is sometimes known as the "pleasure center" of the brain, and also in the amygdala, a critical component of the reactive reward system, which conditions reward responses in association with pleasurable activities.

References

Stahl SM. *Stahl's essential psychopharmacology*, fourth edition. New York, NY: Cambridge University Press; 2013.

Stahl SM, **Grady MM**. *Stahl's illustrated substance use and impulsive disorders*. New York, NY: Cambridge University Press; 2012.

QUESTION TWO

Impulsivity is hypothesized to be related to the _____, while compulsivity is hypothesized to be related to the _____.

A. Amygdala, ventral striatum

B. Ventral striatum, amygdala

C. Dorsal striatum, ventral striatum

D. Ventral striatum, dorsal striatum

Answer to Question Two

The correct answer is D.

Choice	Peer answers
Amygdala, ventral striatum	18%
Ventral striatum, amygdala	11%
Dorsal striatum, ventral striatum	26%
Ventral striatum, dorsal striatum	46%

Impulsivity and compulsivity can perhaps be best differentiated by how they both fail to control responses: impulsivity as the inability to stop initiating actions, and compulsivity as the inability to terminate ongoing actions. Impulsivity and compulsivity are hypothetically neurobiological drives that are "bottom-up," with impulsivity coming from the ventral striatum, compulsivity coming from the dorsal striatum, and different areas of prefrontal cortex acting "top-down" to suppress these drives.

A – Incorrect. The amygdala is involved in reward conditioning and provides input to the striatum, but it is not directly associated with impulsivity. In addition, the dorsal striatum, not the ventral striatum, is associated with compulsivity.

B – Incorrect. Although the ventral striatum is linked to impulsivity, the amygdala is not directly linked to compulsivity.

C – Incorrect. Impulsivity is hypothesized to be related to the ventral striatum, while compulsivity is hypothesized to be related to the dorsal striatum.

D – Correct. Impulsivity is hypothesized to be related to the ventral striatum, while compulsivity is hypothesized to be related to the dorsal striatum.

References
Stahl SM. *Stahl's essential psychopharmacology*, fourth edition. New York, NY: Cambridge University Press; 2013.

QUESTION THREE

73-year-old Laura has had a history of alcohol abuse. When people age, their sensitivity to alcohol increases, as their tolerance decreases, and alcohol takes longer to be metabolized. Many prescribed medications increase the negative effects of alcohol. Laura was recently prescribed desipramine, a tricyclic antidepressant. What are the adverse effects that Laura should be aware of in combining the prescription medication with alcohol, particularly in the first week of treatment?

A. Severe hepatotoxicity with therapeutic doses

B. Increased anticoagulant effects

C. Combined central nervous system (CNS) depression decreases psychomotor performance

D. Masked signs of delirium tremens

Answer to Question Three

The correct answer is C.

Choice	Peer answers
Severe hepatotoxicity with therapeutic doses	7%
Increased anticoagulant effects	1%
Combined central nervous system (CNS) depression decreases psychomotor performance	90%
Masked signs of delirium tremens	2%

A – Incorrect. Acetaminophen at therapeutic doses can result in severe hepatotoxicity in chronic alcoholics, not tricyclic antidepressants.

B – Incorrect. Oral anticoagulants can have decreased anticoagulant effects in chronic alcoholics, not tricyclic antidepressants.

C – Correct. Alcohol abuse, combined with tricyclic antidepressants, such as desipramine, can result in combined CNS depression, resulting in decreased psychomotor performance, especially in the first week of treatment.

D – Incorrect. Beta-adrenergic blockers, when combined with alcohol abuse, may result in masked signs of delirium tremens.

References
Stahl SM, Grady MM. *Stahl's illustrated substance use and impulsive disorders.* New York, NY: Cambridge University Press; 2012.

QUESTION FOUR

Lisa, who is 13, has been staying up later than usual, complaining that she can't sleep. Sometimes during the day, she locks herself in her room for hours, only coming out to use the bathroom. Recently, her mother discovered boxes of hidden cereal, chips, and cookies in her closet. Her mother suspects that Lisa has an eating disorder, but she is not sure if Lisa is vomiting or not, and her weight appears to be normal. Upon psychiatric evaluation, Lisa has negative affect, functional impairment, elevated thin-ideal internalization, and body dissatisfaction. She says she is dieting, but that she is not fasting. Which eating disorder is she at high risk for?

A. Anorexia nervosa

B. Bulimia nervosa

C. Binge-eating disorder

Answer to Question Four

The correct answer is C.

Choice	Peer answers
Anorexia nervosa	9%
Bulimia nervosa	46%
Binge-eating disorder	45%

A – Incorrect. Specific predictive risk factors for anorexia nervosa (AN) include negative affect, functional impairment, and low body mass index (BMI). However, youth who are inherently lean, rather than purposely pursing the thin ideal, are at risk for AN; thus, dieting would not be a specific risk factor for AN. Lisa does not have a low BMI, suggesting that she is not at risk for AN.

B – Incorrect. Specific predictive risk factors for bulimia nervosa (BN) include: thin-ideal internalization, positive thinness expectancy, denial of thin-ideal costs, body dissatisfaction, dieting, negative affect, overeating, fasting, functional impairment, and mental health care. While Lisa suffers from negative affect, overeating, thin-ideal internalization, body dissatisfaction, and functional impairment, she is not fasting.

C – Correct. Specific predictive risk factors for binge-eating disorder (BED) include: elevated thin-ideal internalization, body dissatisfaction, functional impairment, dieting, overeating, negative affect, and mental health care. While negative affect and functional impairment are risk factors for all eating disorders, because Lisa is overeating and hiding her eating habits while openly dieting, she is at high risk for the development of BED.

References

Stahl SM, Grady MM. *Stahl's illustrated substance use and impulsive disorders.* New York, NY: Cambridge University Press; 2012.

Stice, E, Gau JM, Rohde P, Shaw H. Risk factors that predict future onset of each DSM-5 eating disorder. Predictive specificity in high-risk adolescent females. *J Abnorm Psychol* 2017;126(1):38–51.

QUESTION FIVE

A 28-year-old painter presents with a severe drinking problem and you affirm the need for pharmacotherapy. When you suggest naltrexone, the curious artist would like to know how this will help. Which might you use as part of your explanation?

A. Naltrexone blocks mu-opioid receptors to reduce the euphoria you might normally experience with heavy drinking

B. Naltrexone blocks metabotropic glutamate receptors (mGluR) to reduce the euphoria you might normally experience with heavy drinking

C. Naltrexone stimulates mu-opioid receptors to the euphoria you might normally experience with heavy drinking

D. Naltrexone stimulates mGluR receptors to the euphoria you might normally experience with heavy drinking

Answer to Question Five

The correct answer is A.

Choice	Peer answers
Naltrexone blocks mu-opioid receptors to reduce the euphoria you might normally experience with heavy drinking	94%
Naltrexone blocks metabotropic glutamate receptors (mGluR) to reduce the euphoria you might normally experience with heavy drinking	4%
Naltrexone stimulates mu-opioid receptors to the euphoria you might normally experience with heavy drinking	1%
Naltrexone stimulates mGluR receptors to the euphoria you might normally experience with heavy drinking	2%

A – Correct. Blocking mu-opioid receptors might reduce the desire to engage in heavy drinking activity, as doing so will be associated with reduced reward.

B and D – Incorrect. Naltrexone is a mu-opioid antagonist. Mu-opioid receptors theoretically contribute to the "high" or euphoria experienced with heavy drinking, similar to their function in opiate abuse.

C – Incorrect. Blocking mu-opioid receptors, not stimulating them, is the likely mechanism of naltrexone's efficacy.

References
Stahl SM. *Stahl's essential psychopharmacology*, fourth edition. New York, NY: Cambridge University Press; 2013.

Stahl SM, Grady MM. *Stahl's illustrated substance use and impulsive disorders*. New York, NY: Cambridge University Press; 2012.

QUESTION SIX

After seeing a 39-year-old accountant for several years, she has recently disclosed her 10-year prescription opiate addiction to you. She is a quite functional addict, but continues seeking opiates to avoid withdrawal effects. Which of the following might you tell her about her potential for recovery?

A. Opioid receptors can readapt to normal but need a reduction in the amount of opiate exposure over time in order to do so

B. Opioid receptors cannot readapt to normal after severe addiction but can reorganize to nearly full functionality with the aid of permanent pharmacotherapy

Answer to Question Six

The correct answer is A.

Choice	Peer answers
Opioid receptors can readapt to normal but need a reduction in the amount of opiate exposure over time in order to do so	85%
Opioid receptors cannot readapt to normal after severe addiction but can reorganize to nearly full functionality with the aid of permanent pharmacotherapy	15%

A – Correct. The brain's elasticity allows for opioid receptors to readapt to normal after some time of abstinence from drug intake. This may be difficult to tolerate, so reinstituting another opiate, such as methadone, or a partial mu-opiate agonist, such as buprenorphine (in combination with naloxone), may assist the detoxification process.

B – Incorrect.

References

Stahl SM. *Stahl's essential psychopharmacology*, fourth edition. New York, NY: Cambridge University Press; 2013.

Stahl SM, **Grady MM**. *Stahl's illustrated substance use and impulsive disorders*. New York, NY: Cambridge University Press; 2012.

QUESTION SEVEN

A 24-year-old woman with a 6-year history of smoking has decided that she is ready to quit. She is considering nicotine replacement therapy, but is concerned that she may just end up dependent on that instead. Which of the available nicotine replacement therapies carries the highest risk of dependence?

A. Gum

B. Lozenge

C. Nasal spray

D. Oral inhaler

E. Transdermal patch

Answer to Question Seven

The correct answer is C

Choice	Peer answers
Gum	13%
Lozenge	5%
Nasal spray	50%
Oral inhaler	25%
Transdermal patch	7%

A – Incorrect. With the gum, nicotine is absorbed through the mouth; thus, the rate of delivery is slower than with the nasal spray.

B – Incorrect. With the lozenge, nicotine is absorbed through the mouth; thus, the rate of delivery is slower than with the nasal spray.

C – Correct. The risk of dependence is related to the rate at which a drug enters and leaves the brain. The nasal spray has the fastest nicotine delivery of all nicotine replacement therapies and thus carries the highest risk of dependence.

D – Incorrect. Although nicotine is administered with an oral inhaler, it is absorbed in the mouth as opposed to in the lungs.

E – Incorrect. The transdermal patch slowly and steadily delivers nicotine (over 16 or 24 hours), reducing the risk of dependence.

References

Physician's desk reference. Montvale, NJ: Thomson PDR; 2010.

Stahl SM, Grady MM. *Stahl's illustrated substance use and impulsive disorders*. New York, NY: Cambridge University Press; 2012.

QUESTION EIGHT

Mary is a 33-year-old woman with alcohol use disorder. She consumes several drinks a day nearly every day of the week and has recently had her two children removed from her care. She is motivated to attempt to stop drinking in order to get her children back. She previously attempted to quit cold turkey and on her own, and ended up in the emergency room with severe withdrawal symptoms. Considering these factors, would she be a good candidate for reduced-risk drinking as a goal?

A. Yes

B. No

Answer to Question Eight

The correct answer is B.

Choice	Peer answers
Yes	38%
No	62%

A – Incorrect. Because this patient has a history of severe alcohol withdrawal symptoms, she would not be a good candidate for reduced-risk drinking as a goal. In addition, if she does not stop drinking, it is less likely that she will be able to have the children returned to her care.

B – Correct. Reduced-risk drinking as a goal is controversial. However, some patients will not agree to abstinence as a goal. For these patients, it can still be beneficial to work with them to reduce their drinking. Reduced-risk drinking may be a better goal for patients with less severe problems drinking, including at-risk drinkers. The strategy for achieving reduced-risk drinking for patients with alcohol use disorder involves agreeing on a plan. Give patients a choice in the goal if possible – this allows them to take part in decisions affecting their lives and also gives them more responsibility in the outcome. Some sample guidelines for reduced-risk drinking include the "three As": avoid having more than one drink in 1 hour; avoid drinking patterns (same people, same places, same time of day); and avoid drinking to deal with problems.

Contraindications for reduced-risk drinking (as opposed to abstinence) include: existing conditions that would be exacerbated by alcohol, use of disulfiram or other agents contraindicated with alcohol, history of failed attempts with reduced-risk drinking, pregnancy or breastfeeding, and a history of severe alcohol withdrawal symptoms. For patients who should pursue abstinence but refuse, one may try to have them agree to a trial period of abstinence and a trial period of reduced-risk drinking; it can be beneficial to use a written contract.

References

Ambrogne JA. Reduced-risk drinking as a treatment goal: what clinicians need to know. *J Subst Abuse Treatment* 2002;22(1):45–53.

Stahl SM. *Stahl's essential psychopharmacology*, fourth edition. New York, NY: Cambridge University Press; 2013.

Stahl SM, Grady MM. *Stahl's illustrated substance use and impulsive disorders*. New York, NY: Cambridge University Press; 2012.

QUESTION NINE

Clara is at a party with some friends and decides to try "Molly." She was told that "Molly" is the pure form of Ecstasy (3,4-methylenedioxymetamphetamine), lacking many of the harmful additives that can be found in Ecstasy. Upon taking the pill, Clara notices that while she is in a state of excited delirium, she has a nosebleed, she is sweating profusely, and she feels nauseous. She is disoriented, and wonders why she is feeling so horrible after taking the pure form of the drug. Her symptoms are most likely attributed to:

A. A synthetic cathinone, such as methylone

B. Caffeine

C. Methamphetamine

Answer to Question Nine

The correct answer is A.

Choice	Peer answers
A synthetic cathinone, such as methylone	68%
Caffeine	3%
Methamphetamine	29%

A – Correct. While "Molly" is the pure crystal powder form of 3,4-methylenedioxymetamphetamine (MDMA), and lacks the harmful additives commonly found in MDMA, such as caffeine and methamphetamine, the compounds are replaced by dangerous synthetic cathinones, such as methylone. Synthetic cathinones can cause nosebleeds, paranoia, hallucinations, nausea, sweating, panic attacks, and even death.

B and C – Incorrect.

References
Baumann MH. Awash in a sea of 'bath salts': implications for biomedical research and public health. *Addiction* 2014;109(10):1577–9.

QUESTION TEN

Peter is a 17-year-old student who has been using spice (synthetic cannabinoid) over the past year. Synthetic cannabinoids such as spice may be associated with an increased risk of psychosis compared to natural marijuana because they:

A. Do not contain cannabidiol

B. Are full rather than partial agonists

C. A and B

D. Neither A nor B

Answer to Question Ten

The correct answer is C.

Choice	Peer answers
Do not contain cannabidiol	9%
Are full rather than partial agonists	20%
A and B	60%
Neither A nor B	11%

A – Partially correct. Spice use may cause recurrence or exacerbation of pre-existing psychotic symptoms, with studies suggesting a possible three-times increased risk of subsequent psychosis. One factor that may explain why this is seen with spice but not generally with natural marijuana is that natural marijuana contains cannabidiol, which is thought to have antipsychotic properties. In contrast, synthetic cannabinoids do not contain cannabidiol.

B – Partially correct. Unlike natural marijuana, which is a partial agonist at the cannabinoid 1 (CB1) receptor, synthetic cannabinoids are full agonists at CB1. Therefore, they can potentially lead to excessive stimulation of the receptor. In addition, synthetic cannabinoids bind to the CB1 receptor with 800-times greater affinity than natural marijuana.

C – Correct (A and B).

D – Incorrect (neither A nor B).

References

Loeffler G, Hurst D, Penn A, Yung K. Spice, bath salts, and the U.S. military: the emergence of synthetic cannabinoid receptor agonists and cathinones in the U.S. Armed Forces. *Milit Med* 2012;177(9):1041–8.

Seely KA, Lapoint J, Moran JH, Fattore L. Spice drugs are more than harmless herbal blends: a review of the pharmacology and toxicology of synthetic cannabinoids. *Progr Neuropsychopharmacol Biol Psychiatry* 2012;39(2):234–43.

Woo TM, Hanley JR. "How high do they look?": identification and treatment of common ingestions in adolescents. *J Pediatr Health Care* 2013;27: 135–44.

QUESTION ELEVEN

Eddie is a 43-year-old man who has a 22-year-old daughter with a history of cocaine addiction. He recently heard about a novel cocaine vaccine that is being studied and would like to know more about it. In describing the cocaine vaccine, you explain that a cocaine-induced "high" is experienced when:

A. At least 47% of dopamine transporters are occupied by cocaine

B. At least 97% of norepinephrine transporters are occupied by cocaine

C. Both of the above

Answer to Question Eleven

The correct answer is A.

Choice	Peer answers
At least 47% of dopamine transporters are occupied by cocaine	55%
At least 97% of norepinephrine transporters are occupied by cocaine	4%
Both of the above	41%

A – Correct. Studies have shown that the "high" associated with cocaine occurs when at least 47% of dopamine transporters in the brain are occupied by cocaine. When the cocaine vaccine is administered, it causes the production of antibodies that then bind to the vaccine. The antibodies produced in response to the vaccine do not cross into the brain; thus, antibody-bound cocaine remains in the periphery and may therefore reduce the percentage of cocaine-occupied dopamine transporters below the 47% threshold needed to induce a high. One potential advantage of the vaccine is that it prevents cocaine from entering the brain without affecting normal dopamine neurotransmission.

B – Incorrect. Although cocaine does bind to the norepinephrine transporter, it is the effects at the dopamine transporter that are primarily responsible for the induced high.

C – Incorrect (both of the above).

References

Maoz A, Hicks MJ, Vallabhjosula S et al. Adenovirus capsid-based anti-cocaine vaccine prevents cocaine from binding to the nonhuman primate CNS dopamine transporter. *Neuropsychopharmacology* 2013;38: 2170–8.

QUESTION TWELVE

A 26-year-old woman develops a dependence on opioids after taking them during her recovery from knee surgery. She attempts to stop using them on her own, but when she does stop or decreases her dose she experiences nausea, muscle aches, sweating, diarrhea, insomnia, and depression. She and her practitioner decide that buprenorphine would be an appropriate treatment strategy. Which of the following is true?

A. The patients should have the buprenorphine implant, Probuphine, inserted immediately

B. The patient should initiate oral buprenorphine while downtitrating her current opioid

C. The patient should be in a mild withdrawal state prior to initiating buprenorphine

D. The patient should complete withdrawal before beginning buprenorphine treatment

Answer to Question Twelve

The correct answer is C.

Choice	Peer answers
The patients should have the buprenorphine implant, Probuphine, inserted immediately	1%
The patient should initiate oral buprenorphine while downtitrating her current opioid	25%
The patient should be in a mild withdrawal state prior to initiating buprenorphine	66%
The patient should complete withdrawal before beginning buprenorphine treatment	8%

A – Incorrect. The implant Probuphine contains buprenorphine, a partial opioid agonist. Probuphine is indicated for the maintenance treatment of opioid dependence in patients who have achieved and sustained prolonged clinical stability on low-to-moderate doses of a transmucosal buprenorphine-containing product (i.e., doses of no more than 8 mg per day of a sublingual tablet). Probuphine is not appropriate for new entrants to treatment and patients who have not achieved and sustained prolonged clinical stability, while being maintained on buprenorphine sublingual 8 mg per day.

B – Incorrect. Buprenorphine is a partial opioid agonist. It has stronger affinity for the mu opioid receptor than other opioids, and thus causes immediate withdrawal if not administered when the patient is already in withdrawal.

C – Correct. Buprenorphine is a partial opioid agonist. It has stronger affinity for the mu-opioid receptor than other opioids, and thus causes immediate withdrawal if not administered when the patient is already in withdrawal. If the patient is already experiencing withdrawal, however, it will relieve those symptoms. Buprenorphine is commonly combined with naloxone in order to reduce its diversion and intravenous abuse.

D – Incorrect.

References
Chavoustie S, Frost M, Snyder O et al. Buprenorphine implants in medical treatment of opioid addiction. *Expert Rev Clin Pharmacol* 2017; 10(8):799–807.

Dodrill CL, **Helmer DA**, **Kosten TR**. Prescription pain medication dependence. *Am J Psychiatry* 2011;168(5):466–71.

Stahl SM, **Grady MM**. *Stahl's illustrated substance use and impulsive disorders*. New York, NY: Cambridge University Press; 2012.

QUESTION THIRTEEN

A 23-year-old woman has recently been diagnosed with binge-eating disorder. Since the age of 16 she has had episodes where she eats far beyond the point of hunger, typically at night and when she is alone. The patient feels very guilty and disgusted with herself about her eating habits; this is reinforced by her family members, who tell her that she is just weak and should have more self-control. Is there evidence to support the idea that individuals can develop an addiction to food?

A. Yes

B. No

Answer to Question Thirteen

The correct answer is A.

Choice	Peer answers
Yes	95%
No	5%

A – Correct. Food has powerful reinforcing effects. The neurobiological basis of eating and appetite is linked not just to the hypothalamus, but also to the connections that hypothalamic circuits make to reward pathways. Following food deprivation, any food will activate reward pathways. However, palatable (i.e., high-fat, high-sugar) foods activate reward pathways more reliably and more potently than do unpalatable foods. Even without food deprivation, highly palatable foods will activate the release of endocannabinoids and ghrelin; this is not true of unpalatable foods.

There is also evidence that the neurobiological changes associated with the progression to compulsive drug use may similarly occur in individuals with compulsive eating behaviors. When exposed to food cues, obese individuals exhibit increased activation, compared to lean individuals, in regions that process palatability. In contrast, obese individuals exhibit decreased activation of reward circuits during actual food consumption. This is analogous to cravings and tolerance in patients with substance use disorders.

Of course, not everyone who is obese has an eating compulsion, because obesity is also related to genetics and to lifestyle factors such as exercise, caloric intake, and the specific content of consumed foods. In fact, studies of brain activation in response to images of food can differentiate between individuals with binge-eating disorder and overweight controls; in particular, differences in activation have been noted in the right ventral striatum.

B – Incorrect (no).

References

Lutter M, Nestler EJ. Homeostatic and hedonic signals interact in the regulation of food intake. *J Nutr* 2009;139(3):629–32.

Monteleone P, Piscitelli F, Scognamiglio P et al. Hedonic eating is associated with increased peripheral levels of ghrelin and the endocannabinoid 2-arachidonoyl-glycerol in healthy humans: a pilot study. *J Clin Endocrinol Metab* 2012;97:E917–24.

Weygandt M, **Schaefer A**, **Schienle A**, **Haynes JD**. Diagnosing different binge–eating disorders based on reward-related brain activation patterns. *Hum Brain Mapping* 2012;33:2135–46.

CHAPTER PEER COMPARISON

For the Substance Use and Impulsive Compulsive Disorders section, the correct answer was selected 68% of the time.

OVERALL PEER COMPARISON

For *Stahl's Self-Assessment Examination in Psychiatry: Multiple Choice Questions for Clinicians, Third Edition*, the correct answer was selected 68% of the time.

OPTIONAL POSTTESTS AND CME CERTIFICATES

Instructions and Study Guide

CME Credit Expires: December 31, 2020.

Posttests will remain available indefinitely, for your personal enrichment.

The optional online posttests with CME credits are available for a fee (waived for NEI members). For participant ease, each chapter has its own posttest and certificate. NOTE: the book as a whole is considered a single CME activity and credits earned must be totaled and submitted as such to other organizations.

To receive a certificate of CME credit or participation:

1. **Complete a chapter posttest:** *available only online at neiglobal. com/CME (under "Book")*

2. **Print the chapter certificate:** *if a score of 70% or more is achieved*

Questions? call 888–535-5600, or email CustomerService@ neiglobal.com

Study guide for online posttests

The posttest questions have been provided below solely as a study tool to prepare for your online submissions. **Posttests can only be submitted online.** If you do not have access to a computer, contact customer service at 888-535-5600.

Basic Neuroscience

1. A signal transduction cascade passes its message from an extracellular first messenger to an intracellular second messenger. In the case of the G-protein-linked systems, the second messenger is a:
   A. Ion
   B. Hormone
   C. Chemical
   D. Kinase enzyme

2. A receptor with four transmembrane regions changes conformation as GABA binds. Which system is this process describing?
   A. Presynaptic transporter
   B. Ligand–gated ion channel
   C. Voltage-sensitive ion channel

3. Which of the following are involved in regulating neurotransmission via excitation–secretion coupling?
   A. Voltage-sensitive sodium channels
   B. Voltage-sensitive calcium channels
   C. Both A and B
   D. Neither A nor B

4. What are the molecular mechanisms of epigenetics?
   A. Molecular gates are opened by acetylation and/or demethylation of histones, allowing transcription factors access to genes, thus activating them.
   B. Molecular gates are opened by deacetylation and/or methylation, allowing transcription factors access to genes, thus activating them
   C. Molecular gates are closed by deacetylation and/or methylation, preventing access of transcription factors to genes, thus silencing them.
   D. A and C

Psychosis and Schizophrenia and Antipsychotics

1. A 21-year-old man has just been diagnosed with schizophrenia. What pattern of cognitive functioning prior to psychosis onset would you be most likely to find?
   A. Normal cognitive functioning during premorbid and prodromal phases
   B. Impaired cognitive functioning that is stable across premorbid and prodromal phases
   C. Impaired cognitive functioning premorbidly with further decline during the prodromal phase

2. A major current hypothesis for the cause of schizophrenia proposes that N-methyl-D-aspartate (NMDA) receptors may be:
   A. Hypofunctional
   B. Hyperfunctional

3. A 34-year-old man is initiated on an atypical antipsychotic for the treatment of schizophrenia. The majority of atypical antipsychotics:
   A. Have higher affinity for dopamine 2 receptors than for serotonin 2A receptors
   B. Have higher affinity for serotonin 2A receptors than for dopamine 2 receptors

4. A 44-year-old woman with schizophrenia has developed tardive dyskinesia after taking haloperidol 15 mg/day for 2 years. Which of the following would be the most appropriate pharmacologic mechanism to manage her tardive dyskinesia?
   A. Antagonism at serotonin 2A receptors
   B. Antagonism of beta adrenergic receptors
   C. Inhibition of vesicular monoamine transporter 2

Unipolar Depression and Antidepressants

1. A patient with major depressive disorder has not responded to two adequate trials of antidepressant monotherapy. Which of the following has the best evidence of efficacy for augmenting antidepressants in patients with inadequate response?
   A. Atypical antipsychotic
   B. Buspirone
   C. Stimulant

2. A 31-year-old married man has been taking an SSRI for his depression. He discloses that although his mood has improved, he is experiencing sexual dysfunction that is affecting his relationship with his wife. What pharmacological treatment option might be appropriate to address his sexual dysfunction?
   A. 5HT2 antagonist
   B. 5HT3 antagonist
   C. 5HT6 antagonist

3. Symptoms of reduced positive affect (depressed mood, anhedonia, loss of energy) are hypothetically more likely to respond to agents that enhance:
   A. Dopamine and possibly norepinephrine
   B. Norepinephrine and possibly serotonin
   C. Serotonin and possibly dopamine

4. Which of the following foods must be avoided by patients taking MAOIs?
   A. Aged cheeses
   B. Bottled beer
   C. Fresh fish
   D. All of the above
   E. None of the above

Bipolar Disorder and Mood Stabilizers

1. Sam is a 31-year-old patient who presents with a major depressive episode. He has previously been hospitalized and treated for a manic episode but is not currently taking any medication. The agents with the strongest evidence of efficacy in bipolar depression are:
   A. Lamotrigine, lithium, quetiapine
   B. Olanzapine–fluoxetine, lurasidone, lamotrigine
   C. Quetiapine, olanzapine–fluoxetine, lurasidone
   D. Lurasidone, lamotrigine, lithium

2. Patricia is a 39-year-old patient with bipolar I disorder. She has been maintained on 1200 mg/day of lithium. She was doing well for a long time and had even been able to lose the weight she had initially gained with lithium. She lost her job as a postal service worker 6 months ago and has been feeling depressed ever since. You augment her with 300 mg/day of quetiapine, but after several weeks she complains of weight gain and wants to change medications. Blockade of which two receptors was most likely responsible for this weight gain induced by quetiapine?
   A. Serotonin 2C and histamine 1
   B. Serotonin 2A and muscarinic 3
   C. Muscarinic 1 and serotonin 6
   D. Dopamine 2 and alpha 1 adrenergic

3. Diane is a 31-year-old patient with bipolar I disorder who frequently exhibits impulsive symptoms of mania including risk-taking and pressured speech during her manic episodes. Compared to a healthy brain, neuroimaging of this patient's brain during a no-go task (designed to test response inhibition) would likely show:
   A. Increased activity in the dorsolateral prefrontal cortex
   B. Increased activity in the orbitofrontal cortex
   C. Decreased activity in the orbitofrontal cortex

4. Steven is a 29-year-old patient with bipolar II disorder who tends to endorse some manic symptoms during depressive episodes. Of the following symptoms, which is the most common sub-syndromal mania symptom in patients during a major depressive episode with mixed features?
   A. Psychomotor agitation
   B. Decreased need for sleep
   C. Inflated self-esteem
   D. Elevated mood
   E. High-risk behavior

Anxiety Disorders and Anxiolytics

1. A 51-year-old male veteran with chronic PTSD has agreed to begin pharmacotherapy for his debilitating symptoms of arousal and anxiety associated with his experiences in Iraq 2 years ago. Which of the following would be appropriate as first-line treatment?
   A. Paroxetine
   B. Paroxetine or lorazepam
   C. Lorazepam or quetiapine
   D. Paroxetine, lorazepam, or quetiapine

2. Which of the following pharmacotherapy options has been theorized as a potential pre-emptive treatment to the development of PTSD?
   A. N-methyl-D-aspartate (NMDA) agonist such as D-cycloserine
   B. Alpha 2 delta ligand such as pregabalin
   C. Beta adrenergic blocker such as propranolol
   D. Benzodiazepine such as diazepam

3. Which of the following drugs can diminish anxiety but does NOT have sedative, hypnotic, anticonvulsant, or musculoskeletal relaxing activity?
   A. Diazepam
   B. Buspirone
   C. Mirtazapine
   D. Haloperidol

Chronic Pain and its Treatment

1. A young man arrives at the emergency room in great pain after receiving a chemical burn during an accident at work. Which primary afferent neurons would have responded to the chemical stimulus to produce nociceptive neuronal activity?
   A. A beta fiber neurons
   B. A delta fiber neurons
   C. C fiber neurons

2. Does the official diagnosis of fibromyalgia require a tender point diagnosis?
   A. Yes
   B. No

3. Which of the following statements is true?
   A. SSRIs may have inconsistent effects on pain because serotonin can both inhibit and facilitate ascending nociceptive signals
   B. SSRIs may worsen pain because serotonin can facilitate but not inhibit ascending nociceptive signals
   C. SSRIs generally alleviate pain because serotonin can inhibit but not facilitate ascending nociceptive signals
   D. SSRIs generally have no effect on pain because serotonin neither facilitates nor inhibits nociceptive signals

Disorders of Sleep and Wakefulness and their Treatment

1. A 52-year-old female patient with shift work disorder exhibits excessive daytime sleepiness that is interfering with her ability to perform duties as a firefighter. She is initiated on armodafinil with good therapeutic response. Modafinil, and its R-enantiomer armodafinil, are hypothesized to promote wakefulness and increase alertness by:
   A. Decreasing norepinephrine
   B. Decreasing hypocretin/orexin
   C. Increasing histamine
   D. All of the above
   E. None of the above

2. Sheila is a 41-year-old woman who recently underwent diagnostic testing for obstructive sleep apnea. Results show that this patient has an apnea–hypopnea index (AHI) of 37. An AHI of 37 is indicative of:
   A. No sleep apnea
   B. Mild sleep apnea
   C. Moderate sleep apnea
   D. Severe sleep apnea

3. A clinician is planning to prescribe eszopiclone for a 51-year-old male patient with insomnia. What is the correct starting dose for this patient?
   A. 0.5 mg/night
   B. 1 mg/night
   C. 2 mg/night
   D. 3 mg/night

4. A 13-year-old male patient has been brought to the clinic by his parents for evaluation. The patient typically sleeps for 11 or more hours a day (yet still exhibits excessive daytime sleepiness), eats excessive amounts of food, and demonstrates disinhibited behaviors. This patient most likely has:
   A. Idiopathic hypersomnia
   B. Narcolepsy without cataplexy
   C. Kleine–Levin syndrome

Attention Deficit Hyperactivity Disorder (ADHD) and its Treatment

1. According to DSM-5 criteria, what is the maximum age threshold for symptom onset when making a diagnosis of attention deficit hyperactivity disorder (ADHD)?
   A. 8
   B. 10
   C. 12
   D. 14

2. Which of the following drugs are transported into neurons via the dopamine transporter?
   A. Amphetamine
   B. Atomoxetine
   C. Methylphenidate
   D. A and B
   E. A, B, and C

3. Aggregate data suggest that, at the class level, the effect size of stimulants is:
   A. Smaller than that of non-stimulants
   B. Approximately the same as that of non-stimulants
   C. Larger than that of non-stimulants

Dementia and Cognitive Function and its Treatment

1. Mike is a 50-year-old accountant with a family history of Alzheimer's disease. He recently had amyloid positron emission tomography (amyloid PET) neuroimaging done and, although he currently exhibits no behavioral symptoms of Alzheimer's disease, Mikes's amyloid PET scans revealed accumulation of beta amyloid protein throughout cortical and limbic areas of his brain. Although much research is yet to be done, data indicate that the normal physiological role of amyloid beta protein may include:
   A. Blood vessel repair functions
   B. Antimicrobial functions
   C. Both of the above

2. Harriet is a 69-year-old patient recently diagnosed with probable Alzheimer's disease. This patient would like to start treatment with a cholinesterase inhibitor; however, she has been a chain smoker for over 50 years and refuses to give up the habit. Which of the following medications would not be appropriate for this patient, given her smoking habit?
   A. Donepezil
   B. Galantamine
   C. Rivastigmine
   D. None of these medications should be prescribed to a patient who smokes
   E. There are no contraindications due to smoking for these medications

3. Pete is a 46-year-old man with progressive amnesic memory loss and cognitive deficits beginning approximately 1 year ago. Neuropsychiatric testing shows moderate cognitive impairment not attributable to any medical or psychiatric condition. Amyloid PET imaging indicates that this patient has amyloid beta protein accumulation in his brain and genetic testing has revealed that he carries an Alzheimer's-associated mutation in the presenilin gene. What would be the most likely diagnosis for this patient according to the National Institute on Aging and Alzheimer's Association 2011 diagnostic criteria for dementia?
   A. Possible Alzheimer's dementia
   B. Probable Alzheimer's dementia with increased level of certainty
   C. Alzheimer's dementia

Substance Use and Impulsive Compulsive Disorders and their Treatment

1. Your 16-year-old son is thrilled when he wins the 100-meter dash in an important high school competition. This "natural high" is most likely associated with inducing dopamine release in his mesolimbic pathway and in his:
   A. Hypothalamus
   B. Amygdala
   C. Hippocampus
   D. Cerebellum
   E. Motor cortex

2. Lisa, who is 13, has been staying up later than usual, complaining that she can't sleep. Sometimes during the day, she locks herself in her room for hours, only coming out to use the bathroom. Recently, her mother discovered boxes of hidden cereal, chips, and cookies in her closet. Her mother suspects that Lisa has an eating disorder, but she is not sure if Lisa is vomiting or not, and her weight appears to be normal. Upon psychiatric evaluation, Lisa has negative affect, functional impairment, elevated thin-ideal internalization, and body dissatisfaction. She says she is dieting, but that she is not fasting. Which eating disorder is she at high risk for?
   A. Anorexia nervosa
   B. Bulimia nervosa
   C. Binge-eating disorder

3. A 28-year-old painter presents with a severe drinking problem and you affirm the need for pharmacotherapy. When you suggest naltrexone, the curious artist would like to know how this will help. Which might you use as part of your explanation?
   A. Naltrexone blocks mu-opioid receptors to reduce the euphoria you might normally experience with heavy drinking
   B. Naltrexone blocks metabotropic glutamate receptors (mGluR) to reduce the euphoria you might normally experience with heavy drinking
   C. Naltrexone stimulates mu-opioid receptors to the euphoria you might normally experience with heavy drinking
   D. Naltrexone stimulates mGluR receptors to the euphoria you might normally experience with heavy drinking

4. Clara is at a party with some friends and decides to try "Molly." She was told that "Molly" is the pure form of Ecstasy (3,4-methylenedioxymetamphetamine), lacking many of the harmful additives that can be found in Ecstasy. Upon taking the pill, Clara notices that while she is in a state of excited delirium, she has a nosebleed, she is sweating profusely, and she feels nauseous. She is disoriented, and wonders why she is feeling so horrible after taking the pure form of the drug. Her symptoms are most likely attributed to:
   A. A synthetic cathinone, such as methylone
   B. Caffeine
   C. Methamphetamine

INDEX

Index

Index